Vernon Coleman trained as a doctor and
practised as a GP for ten years. Now a
full-time author, he has written over
thirty books which have been translated
into eleven languages and sold all round
the world. He broadcasts frequently on
both TV and radio and writes regularly
for a number of major newspapers and
magazines.

Also by Vernon Coleman

BODYPOWER
ADDICTS AND ADDICTIONS
LIFE WITHOUT TRANQUILLISERS
THE PATIENT'S COMPANION

and published by Corgi Books

Dr Vernon Coleman's

GUIDE TO
ALTERNATIVE
MEDICINE

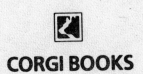

CORGI BOOKS

DR VERNON COLEMAN'S
GUIDE TO ALTERNATIVE MEDICINE

A CORGI BOOK 0 552 13100 8

First publication in Great Britain

PRINTING HISTORY
Corgi edition published 1988

Copyright © 1988 Dr Vernon Coleman

This book is set in 10/11 pt Cheltenham
by Colset Private Limited, Singapore.

Corgi Books are published by Transworld Publishers Ltd.,
61–63 Uxbridge Road, Ealing, London W5 5SA, in Australia
by Transworld Publishers (Australia) Pty. Ltd., 15–23 Helles
Avenue, Moorebank, NSW 2170, and in New Zealand by
Transworld Publishers (N.Z.) Ltd., Cnr. Moselle and
Waipareira Avenues, Henderson, Auckland.

Made and printed in Great Britain by
The Guernsey Press Co. Ltd., Guernsey, Channel Islands.

Contents

Foreword

by Professor Harold Oaks, FSAMP, PCMT

As President of the College of Medical Therapists and Visiting Professor of Holistic Medicine at the University of Rome I am delighted to have the opportunity to write this foreword to Dr Vernon Coleman's honest and forthright book on the subject of alternative medicine.

During recent years there have been many advances in the various sciences which make up the world of alternative medicine. It is now without doubt extremely difficult for patients and practitioners alike to keep up to date or to differentiate between those therapeutic advances which are worthwhile and important and those which are of lesser value.

I believe that Dr Coleman's book will become a classic and will be welcomed by all those who have an interest in this fascinating subject.

H. Oaks

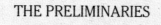

THE PRELIMINARIES

1 The demand for alternative medicine is fired and fuelled by disenchantment with orthodox medicine

The popularity of alternative, or complementary, medicine has increased rapidly in the last few years. All around the world the number of people practising acupuncture, herbalism, hypnotherapy and other complementary forms of medicine increases annually. In just about every developed country in the world millions of people regularly seek help from alternative practitioners.

There are a number of different reasons why people consult alternative practitioners. But by far the commonest reason is a dissatisfaction with what orthodox medicine has to offer. Patients are frightened by the high incidence of side effects known to be associated with the use of modern drugs and surgical techniques; they are annoyed by the lack of time and courtesy offered to them by clinicians of all kinds; and they are attracted by the promises of a sympathetic manner and of risk-free therapies that are associated with alternative practitioners.

There is little doubt in my mind that the dissatisfaction with orthodox medicine is well-founded. There is now ample evidence available to show that medical-school-trained practitioners are often more interested in their research programmes than in the welfare of their patients, and more interested in the science of medicine than the art of healing.

In recent years numerous books and research articles have been published which have shown that too often doctors do more harm than good and that the affection shown by doctors for

11

high-technology medicine is often misplaced. Two of my own earliest books, *The Medicine Men* and *Paper Doctors*, described some of the specific problems associated with twentieth-century medicine in close detail.

In the nineteenth century the medical profession made enormous strides forward. At the beginning of that century life expectancy was low and millions of babies and young children never grew to adulthood. Diseases such as smallpox, typhoid, cholera and tuberculosis devastated whole communities. By the end of the century things had changed dramatically. Life expectancy had improved enormously and infants stood a much better chance of living to childhood and even adulthood. Improvements in public health facilities, in housing regulations, in food supplies and in agricultural policies had all helped to ensure that people had more to eat, better homes to live in, cleaner water to drink and greater protection against disease and infection.

By the start of the twentieth century the future looked bright. The drugs industry was just developing and surgical skills were being honed to new, high standards. Anyone alive at the start of this century would have felt confident that the medical profession would bloom and that in future people would lead longer and healthier lives.

But things haven't quite worked out as expected.

Within the last twenty years more money has been spent on medical care and research than had been spent in the whole of the rest of man's history on Earth. Health care has become one of the world's largest and fastest growing industries. And yet we have very little to show for all the money and effort that has been expended.

Despite the fact that most individual doctors remain committed to caring for the sick and the infirm, medicine has sunk into a slough and there has been almost no improvement in either the quality or quantity of life enjoyed in the developed countries of the world.

Medicine has become full of confusions and paradoxes. Doctors keep alive a greater proportion of our over-65-year-olds and over-75-year-olds. But at the same time there has been an increase in the number of people dying in their 30s and 40s. The expenditure on health care has rocketed but the statistics show that people are now more likely to fall ill than they were a generation ago. The number of doctors goes up annually. But whenever doctors go on strike the death rate goes down.

We have richer food supplies and more readily available medicines today than ever before. But all the evidence suggests that

12

people were never healthier than during the ravages of the Second World War. Governments claim to recognize the value of preventive medicine and yet half the adult population and a third of the child population take some form of medicament every day.

During the last quarter of a century we have developed remarkably sophisticated machinery for our hospitals, and yet cancers, immune disorders and allergy problems become commoner every day. We now have specialist coronary care units for heart-attack victims, and yet more people than ever are dying of heart disease. Young people are bigger and stronger than their ancestors, and yet the number of patients suffering from diabetes is doubling every decade. More and more people are living in air-conditioned, centrally heated buildings and yet infections still kill millions. We have more drugs than ever before and yet we are now all terrified of AIDS. We have more surgeons and more operating theatres than at any other time, and yet there are enormous waiting lists for essential surgery. New procedures and drugs are tested more extensively than ever before, and yet the incidence of doctor-induced disease continues to rise. We have the technology to prevent unwanted pregnancies, and yet the demand for abortions never stops growing. Medicine has never been more sophisticated, and yet patients have never been more dissatisfied. Doctors have never tried harder and never been less well loved.

Most dramatic of all are these simple facts: overall life expectancy in the developed world hasn't changed in the last twenty years while life expectancy at the age of 45 hasn't changed since the beginning of the century.

Orthodox medicine has been tried and been found wanting. It is hardly surprising that alternative medicine becomes more popular month by month.

2   Quacks and charlatans – 1980s style

The boom years of alternative medicine have seen the development of a vast number of medical specialities. Some, such as acupuncture, are ancient. Others, such as biochemistry, are relatively modern; some are symptomatic (homoeopathy), others are designed to improve the overall health of the individual (naturopathy); some are based on mental powers (meditation), others are purely physical (reflexology); some are clearly and unarguably interventionist (herbalism) while others encourage the individual to use his own powers (mindpower). Some techniques are logical and physical (massage), while others are irrational and illogical (radionics and iridology).

Some are old, some are new and some are merely modern variations on old-fashioned themes.

The boom years have seen an explosion in the number of practitioners offering alternative medicine services. Walk through any decent-sized town and you'll find rows of brass plates advertising the services of hypnotherapists, acupuncturists, herbalists and osteopaths. Let your fingers walk idly through the telephone directory and you'll find advertisements for homoeopaths, chiropractors, hydrotherapists, kinaesthesiologists and a hundred and one other impressive-sounding specialities.

For the individual patient wanting to take advantage of the services offered by today's alternative practitioners there is one enormous problem: how to differentiate between the well-qualified practitioner and the out-and-out quack.

Surprising though it may seem, there are few laws about just who can or cannot practise alternative medicine. And there are no laws to prevent individuals who are after a quick buck from setting them-

14

selves up as training establishments or colleges and offering diplomas by post to students prepared to part with the appropriate fee.

It is possible for someone with absolutely no medical training to leave a factory or office job on Friday evening and set up shop as a hypnotherapist or herbalist on Monday morning.

You can buy a brass plate and a leather couch, rent a room and set up shop wherever you fancy your chances. And if you feel that your status will be helped by a diploma or two, or a few impressive-sounding qualifications, then you can buy all the qualifications you need as easily as you can buy a brass plate or a consulting couch.

There are practitioners offering their services today who couldn't pass O-level biology. There are practitioners in all alternative medical specialities who know virtually nothing about anatomy or physiology. There are thousands of practitioners around who are a positive menace and a danger to the health of their patients.

If you feel that I'm exaggerating then look once again at the Foreword to this book. It was written by Professor Harold Oaks, President of the College of Medical Therapists, Visiting Professor of Holistic Medicine at the University of Rome and a Fellow of the Society of Alternative Medicine Practitioners.

Professor Oaks may sound well qualified but in fact Harold is a friendly toad who lives in my woodshed. As far as I know he has no qualifications of any kind. There is no such thing as the College of Medical Therapists. There is no Professor of Holistic Medicine at the University of Rome. And there is no Society of Alternative Medicine Practitioners.

Remember Professor H. Oaks next time you see a brass plate or visiting card or newspaper advertisement for an apparently well-qualified acupuncturist, hypnotherapist, osteopath, herbalist or homoeopath. There are no officially recognized qualifications for such practitioners. There is no official list of careful and well-trained practitioners. There are many colleges and teaching establishments and registration authorities which claim that they are 'official'. But there is, I fear, an excellent chance that the apparently well-qualified practitioner who advertises in your local newspaper is no better trained and no better qualified than the toad who lives in my woodshed.

3 Alternative practitioners are too uncritical

Practitioners – and patients – who favour alternative medicine are often, rightly, critical of orthodox medical practitioners.

But practitioners – and patients – who favour alternative medicine hardly ever apply the same critical eye to their own practices and beliefs.

During the last ten years or so I have read thousands of books and articles written by practitioners of such specialities as acupuncture, herbalism, hypnotherapy and homoeopathy. But I have yet to find a book or article written by an alternative medicine practitioner (or patient) which criticizes any aspect of alternative medicine.

Alternative practitioners often complain that orthodox practitioners are dangerous, inconsistent, inefficient, badly trained, greedy and unscientific. But these criticisms are all, in varying degrees, true of aspects of alternative medicine. And those who support alternative medicine do not, in my view, do their cause any good by highlighting the virtues of their favourite speciality while failing to take note of the problems and shortcomings associated with that speciality.

The truth, of course, is that much alternative medicine is good and useful. But it is also true that much alternative medicine is worthless and dangerous.

Those who support alternative medicine do their cause no good at all by trying to disguise this fact.

4 The desperate need for research

One of the criticisms commonly levelled at those who practise ortho-dox medicine is that new techniques and new drugs are not properly tested before being made available to the general public. There is more than a little truth in this accusation.

But there is, I fear, a far greater shortage of reliable, responsible research work in the field of alternative medicine.

While preparing this book I desperately searched through the world's medical and scientific journals for scientific papers proving that alternative medicine really works. On the whole I searched in vain. Very few research projects of any quality have been undertaken and very few papers of any quality have been published.

Those who practise alternative medicine have a number of excuses for this sad state of affairs.

First, they say that it is not possible to test alternative medicine in the same way that it is possible to test orthodox medicine. I fear, however, that this defence simply does not stand up under scrutiny. The truth is that it would be possible to test the efficacy of any alternative medicine speciality. Any half-way qualified research scientist would be able to plan a series of useful and valid research projects.

Secondly, they say that there is not enough money in alternative medicine to pay for trials to be done. This is a weak and entirely indefensible argument. The practice of alternative medicine is now very big business. Many practitioners make an excellent living out of osteopathy, hypnotherapy and chiropractic. You only have to look at the brass plates in and around Harley Street in London (the world's most exclusive area for expensive practitioners) to see just how successful some of Britain's alternative practitioners are. Moreover, there are also many large companies making huge amounts of money out of the sale of herbal products, vitamin preparations and other alternative therapies.

Thirdly, those who do not want to conduct proper research trials say that there is no need for scientific evidence because they know that their treatments work. That really is a pathetic argument. Anyone who has studied the powerful placebo effect will know that when a practitioner offers a patient a treatment then there is an excellent chance that the very act of offering the treatment will be enough to induce recovery. Give one hundred patients in pain a sugar pill and half of them will get better.

Finally, it is argued that no proper trials have been organized because the drug companies and the orthodox doctors are not interested in organizing any trials or starting any research programmes. What a strange argument! That is rather like Hoffman La Roche saying that their latest drug hasn't been tested because Wyeth Laboratories wouldn't organize the research! It's like the nuclear fuel industry expecting the electricity industry to do its research work for it.

5 Despite claims to the contrary alternative medicine can be dangerous

Those who practise alternative medicine often claim that their treatments are entirely safe. This is not true. There are a number of very real dangers associated with all types of alternative medicine.

First, there are the intrinsic dangers associated with alternative therapies even when they are practised competently. In January 1986, for example, the *British Medical Journal* contained a report of several patients whose spinal cords had been damaged by osteopathic manipulation. Other reports have shown that there are real hazards with just about all alternative practices. The most hazardous speciality is probably herbalism and further details of the type of problems associated with herb therapy are described briefly on page 101.

Secondly, there is the very real risk that because of a poor training an alternative practitioner will make an incorrect diagnosis and treat a patient improperly. For example, in one well-documented case a 22-year-old woman died of tuberculosis after being treated with Epsom salts, herbs and a fruit diet by a homoeopath who thought she was constipated. There is, in addition, the risk that by using apparently scientific diagnostic aids, such as Kirlian photography and iridology, a practitioner will persuade his patients that he is capable of making sound diagnostic decisions.

Thirdly, there is the equally real risk that a treatment offered by an alternative practitioner will interact dangerously with a treatment offered simultaneously by an orthodox practitioner. Prescribed drugs and herbal products are, for example, particularly likely to produce a dangerous response. In theory patients should always tell their doctors when seeing alternative practitioners (and vice versa). In practice, however, many patients are too embarrassed to be honest and continue to put themselves at risk by continuing with two different treatments at the same time.

Fourthly, there is the problem that alternative practitioners are not usually available at night or at weekends. This means that in an emergency the patient of such a practitioner will be left to fend for himself.

6 Mix and match orthodox and alternative

In the past those who have written about alternative medicine have fallen into two clearly defined categories. On the one hand there have been those who have dismissed all alternative remedies as irrational and irrelevant. On the other hand there have been those who have praised and supported all aspects of alternative medicine without reservation or criticism. Some doctors have claimed that all alternative practitioners are ignorant and useless. Some alternative therapists have claimed that they have all the answers to all medical problems.

I believe that the truth lies somewhere in between these two extremes. Some forms of alternative medicine are dangerous and useless, other alternative solutions are safe and effective. Some alternative practitioners are rogues, anxious only to make money out of their patients; others are honest, honourable and responsible. Some disorders are best treated by alternative practitioners while others need the attention of orthodox medical practitioners. Patients should, I believe, be encouraged to use a mixture of all the available regimes, both orthodox and complementary. The human body responds to many different methods of treatment and in future I would like to see all practitioners aware of this and prepared to combine their energies and skills for the benefit of their patients.

In order to prepare what I believe is the first, honest, unbiased appraisal of all popular forms of alternative medicine I have spoken and written to thousands of patients and practitioners. And I have read thousands of books and articles dealing with specific and general aspects of alternative medicine. Inevitably, in order to keep this book to a manageable length I have had to exclude many of the more

21

esoteric therapies, most of the purely psychological therapies (President Carter's Commission on Mental Health listed no fewer than 140 different forms of psychotherapy), and all of those therapies which are concerned primarily with general inner development.

I have also deliberately omitted from this book details and addresses of organizations and associations which claim to offer training or registration for practitioners. The plain fact is that although there are many organizations which claim to represent alternative practitioners there are no officially recognized organizations and I have found it impossible to differentiate between those associations which can offer a high quality of care and service and those which can only make promises. In Britain, for example, I have found 14 organizations representing acupuncturists, 9 representing herbalists, 15 representing homoeopaths, 19 representing hypnotherapists and 16 representing osteopaths. In the absence of any official, registered list of practitioners or colleges it is impossible to decide which qualifications are worth respecting and which are worthless.

I have, therefore, formulated a few basic guidelines of my own for readers who want to take advantage of the skills offered by alternative therapists.

1   Orthodox medical practitioners are undoubtedly the best equipped to deal with acute conditions. In an emergency of any kind I suggest that patients call their own general practitioners or visit their nearest hospital.

2   Where there is doubt about a diagnosis then a visit to an orthodox medical professional is essential. Alternative therapists are poor at making diagnoses and can, on occasions, make very serious errors.

3   Alternative therapists are often very good at dealing with specific problems. (For example, osteopaths are good at dealing with bad backs; acupuncturists are good at dealing with persistent pain.) The information available in the A to Z section of this book will help you decide what conditions are best treated by which specialists.

4   By and large, alternative practitioners are particularly good at dealing with chronic or persistent medical problems. There are, for example, practitioners who are good at dealing with the following problems:

   •   musculo-skeletal problems such as backache, arthritis and rheumatism

- persistent pain of all kinds
- allergies
- chronic, persistent or recurrent infections such as cystitis which cannot be treated effectively by orthodox practitioners
- circulatory problems such as high blood pressure
- an inability to relax or get to sleep at night
- general tiredness
- anxieties and all stress-related disorders

5 Never visit an alternative practitioner who advertises. The best organizations and associations of therapists do not allow their members to advertise at all. The hypnotherapist or homoeopath who advertises in your local newspaper could well have bought his diploma over the counter or undergone a brief and woefully inadequate correspondence course in the subject.

6 The best way to choose a good local practitioner is by word of mouth. Ask your friends and relatives if they know of a good acupuncturist or hypnotherapist. And don't be afraid to ask your family doctor or general practitioner for advice. Recent research has shown that the majority of doctors do not disapprove of their patients seeking help from alternative therapists – indeed, they often welcome it. Your own family doctor will probably know which local alternative therapists are reliable and honest and which are incompetent and unscrupulous.

7 A good alternative practitioner will practise from clean and properly equipped premises. Never visit a practitioner who works in a back bedroom or living room.

THE A TO Z OF ALTERNATIVE MEDICINE

ACUPRESSURE

The background

Some historians believe that when acupuncture (q.v.) meridians were first mapped practitioners did not use sharp needles but used their fingers instead. Furthermore they believe that the needles were only introduced to give the therapist the feeling that he was 'doing' something – and to give a certain amount of status to the practitioner.

Acupuncture with fingers rather than needles is called 'acupressure' and has been a recognized modern therapy for half a century or so.

As with acupuncture the aim is restore the flow of energy along a meridian pathway, stimulating the flow when there is a blockage and bringing energy into the system when a meridian is empty.

To make a diagnosis

Acupressure is normally only used for the treatment of specific conditions where the diagnosis is clear to both the patient and the practitioner.

The provision of treatment

In practice acupressure is a mixture of acupuncture and massage. It is also similar to shiatsu. The acupressure therapist presses hard on specific parts of the patient's body using only his or her fingertips.

Different acupressure therapists use different acupressure points and there doesn't seem to be a great deal of agreement between therapists about the best places to stimulate in order to relieve specific symptoms.

There are several important practical points about acupressure.

First, acupressure is a useful self-help technique. You can experiment with acupressure on different parts of your body and discover your own most effective acupressure points. Medical scientists have shown that a stimulating massage just about anywhere on the human body can help produce the body's own pain-relieving hormones – the endorphins – and I strongly suspect that the site you choose is far less important than the way you do the massage.

Secondly, acupressure should be done with the fingertips. And it is important to press quite hard. You need to exert a downward pressure of about ten pounds. You can get a 'feel' of what this means by pressing down on your bathroom scales.

Thirdly, the most effective acupressure points seem to be on or around the head and neck. By using finger massage at the top of the spine, on the centre of the cheeks, on the outer edges of the eyes and on the centre of the forehead between the eyes it is possible to relieve a wide range of symptoms. Another acupressure point that is well worth trying is the one in the fleshy web that lies between the thumbs and forefingers of both hands. Massaging the acupressure point here is said to be particularly useful for relieving pain.

Research

Acupressure has not yet been subjected to clinical trials of the type that have been done with acupuncture.

Qualifications and training for acupressure

I know of no official training schools and no formal qualifications for would be acupressure therapists. There are, however, undoubtedly small colleges which do provide acupressure diplomas to their students.

Dangers

Since acupressure is a non-invasive, gentle therapy it is extremely unlikely that any patient could ever be damaged by acupressure treatment.

The uses of acupressure

Acupressure is said to be very useful for the temporary relief of distress or pain. It is widely used for headaches, toothache, backache, muscle pains, arthritis and menstrual cramps. It is also used to relieve sleeplessness, diarrhoea, constipation and depression.

ACUPUNCTURE

The background

Acupuncture is one of the oldest forms of medical treatment and can be traced back thousands of years. Archaeologists have even found bronze acupuncture needles which, they claim, suggest that acupuncture was practised during the Bronze Age – two or three thousand years BC.

There are a number of theories about just how acupuncture started. One of the most colourful is that primitive warriors, injured by enemy arrows, discovered that although the wounds they received were painful their chronic muscle and bone pains disappeared in the weeks after injury. They decided that there was a link between their injuries and the disappearance of their chronic pains and, so the story goes, learned to prick themselves with sharp arrow heads in order to get rid of disabling pains.

Whatever the truth may be about the origins of acupuncture there is very little doubt that it was in China where acupuncture was first used widely.

The traditional Chinese believed that human life is activated by an internal energy force which they called 'chi' and that as long as this internal energy force is allowed to flow freely around the body then diseases will be kept at bay.

The theory upon which the practice of acupuncture is founded is that the human body contains twelve main meridians or channels along which this vital internal energy can flow. When one or more of these meridians are blocked in some way then the flow of energy is impeded and the individual will become ill.

The practice of acupuncture is built upon the claim that there are a number of specific points on the human body which can be regarded as entrances or exits for this internal energy force. As long ago as the fourteenth century Chinese doctors had identified 657 acupuncture points. Today over a thousand acupuncture points have been identified.

To make a diagnosis

Before attempting to free the flow of energy the acupuncturist must first decide what is wrong with his patient. Only by making an accurate diagnosis can the acupuncturist decide precisely where the blockage is – and where the needles must be inserted.

The skilled acupuncturist will make his diagnosis in a number of ways. He will look at his patient, study his skin tone, breathing rate and other signs; he will listen to the tone and timbre of his voice and he will perform a careful, painstaking physical examination. One of the most important parts of the physical examination is the taking of the pulse. Unlike Western doctors, practitioners of Chinese medicine recognize twelve different pulses, all palpable on the wrists of the patient's hands, but providing a good deal of information about the condition of the internal organs.

The provision of treatment

Once the diagnosis has been made the acupuncturist can then try to clear the blocked meridians – and restore the flow of energy – by inserting special needles into the skin at special predetermined acupuncture points.

In ancient China acupuncture needles were made of gold, silver, wood, bamboo or bone. These days they are usually made of stainless steel or copper. The needles vary in length from a fraction of an inch to 7 in. Their diameter is usually $1/17,000$ in or $1/18,000$ in. Obviously, it is important that the needles be properly sterilized between the treatment of each patient.

Although choosing the correct acupuncture point is vitally important it isn't just the site of insertion that determines the type of treatment that is given. The angle at which the needle is inserted, the way it is moved around by twirling, pushing or pulling and the time it is left in position will all affect the final results. Some modern acupuncturists use electrical stimulation to activate the acupuncture needles. Using electrical stimulation enables the acupuncturist to control the type of treatment he gives without constantly touching and twirling the needles.

Occasionally, as an alternative to using needles, acupuncturists will use a technique known as moxibustion. This involves drying and shredding leaves of the Chinese wormwood plant and then burning the shredded leaves (known as moxa wool) directly over an acupuncture point. Moxibustion, a type of localized hot poultice remedy which applies heat to a specific point on the body, can be used either alone or together with traditional needle acupuncture. Moxibustion is said to 'tone' and 'supplement' the body's vital energy flow and acupuncturists recommend it for chronic ailments such as arthritis.

There is one other form of treatment used occasionally by some modern acupuncturists, and that is 'ear acupuncture'. Those who practise this type of acupuncture believe that by puncturing specific parts of the ear they can treat disorders affecting any part of the body. The ear, they claim, is a miniature body map.

Ear acupuncture is particularly popular among acupuncturists who treat patients wanting to lose weight or give up smoking. Sometimes a small staple will be left in the ear and the patient will be encouraged to touch it (and stimulate it) when he feels the desire to eat or to smoke.

Just how acupuncture works is something of a mystery. Western scientists have argued that it may work by blocking channels which normally transmit pain impulses or by stimulating the body to produce endorphins – its own, natural, internal painkilling hormones. Traditional acupuncturists dismiss these theories as too simplistic and simply argue that it isn't necessary to understand how acupuncture works in order to benefit from it.

Research

There seems little doubt that acupuncture does often work well. Back in 1974 four American surgeons reported that they had treated over three hundred patients in and around the New York area by acupuncture. The surgeons stated that in over three-quarters of the cases they had found that acupuncture is one of the most effective treatments available for arthritis, neuralgia and other skeletomuscular pains.

Two doctors writing in the *Canadian Anaesthetists Society Journal* in the same year reported that when used as an anaesthetic acupuncture had a success rate of up to 90 per cent and concluded that 'the effectiveness of acupuncture can no longer be doubted'.

By 1979 acupuncture had been so widely tested and tried that at a meeting of medical representatives from all six of the World Health Organization's regions it was concluded that 'the sheer weight of evidence demands that it must be taken seriously as a clinical procedure of considerable value'. The World Health Organization subsequently condemned doctors for failing to accept acupuncture as a useful medical technique, arguing that the antagonistic attitude of many doctors and other health professionals has proved a major obstacle and has hindered the acceptance of acupuncture.

Since 1980 the number of published papers about acupuncture has continued to grow – indeed, there are probably as many scientific papers about acupuncture as there are about all other forms of alternative medicine put together.

Not all the papers that have been published have confirmed the usefulness of acupuncture. For example, in 1982 the *Journal of the Royal Society of Medicine* in London published a paper entitled 'Effects of Acupuncture in Bronchial Asthma' that had been written by a physiologist, an anaesthetist and a pharmacologist from Sri Lanka. After studying twenty patients the scientists concluded that acupuncture has nothing more than a placebo effect in bronchial asthma. Other papers have shown that acupunture is not, for example, particularly useful in helping patients to stop smoking.

But despite the existence of these critical research papers the fact remains that there is now a considerable amount of evidence to show that acupuncture *can* help many patients – particularly patients suffering from pain. There are few, if any, orthodox forms of treatment that are not the subject of constant argument and debate. And it is hardly surprising that scientists are still uncertain about the precise value of acupuncture.

Qualifications and training for acupuncturists

The training programme to become an acupuncturist can take anything from two days to three years – the shorter courses being particularly popular among registered medical practitioners who want to offer acupuncture to their patients. Obviously, therefore, the quality of care offered by acupuncturists varies considerably. I know of no safe and certain way to differentiate between skilled and unskilled acupuncturists. I suggest that patients intending to visit acupuncturists read and follow the general advice given on page 22.

Dangers

Despite claims to the contrary problems can occur when acupuncture is performed. For example, in 1977 in Birmingham an outbreak of hepatitis was traced back to an acupuncturist who had been using dirty needles. And at a meeting between the British Medical Association's working party on alternative therapies and the British Medical Acupuncture Society, Dr Virginia Camp, a consultant rheumatologist and chairman of the Acupuncture Society, reported that a patient who was having treatment for back pain died of respiratory failure after a needle had punctured a lung.

In a television interview Professor J. Worsley of the College of Traditional Chinese Acupuncture in Leamington Spa, Warwickshire, told me that he knew of patients who had needed to be admitted to mental hospitals after having had thoughtlessly administered acupuncture.

But although there undoubtedly are dangers with acupuncture it is important not to over-emphasize them. When acupuncture is done carefully, in hygienic surroundings, by properly trained acupuncturists, and when the contraindications are not ignored (it is said that acupuncture should not be done when a patient is exhausted, has heart trouble, has just eaten, or is bleeding) then the risks are minimal. Dr David Bresler, the Director of the Pain Treatment Center at UCLA Medical School, says that a list of over 3,000 patients (who had between them received 500,000 'needlings') did not show a single case of damage or infection.

According to many experts the dangers that do exist would disappear if the orthodox medical profession would accept acupuncture as a proper medical speciality. The World Health Organization has claimed that it is because doctors have remained sceptical about acupuncture that the practice of this medical speciality has been infiltrated by unscrupulous and ill-informed practitioners who have preyed on patients who are anxious for help but who don't know how to obtain useful, safe and effective treatment.

The uses of acupuncture

Acupuncture works best in long term conditions and in conditions that are reversible. It is not a good treatment for major infections or for cancer.

In 1979 the World Health Organization listed a number of diseases that could be helped by acupuncture.

The important word is 'could' – not every patient with a disease on this list will be cured by acupuncture treatment.

The list includes the following disorders:

Upper respiratory tract
    acute sinusitis

33

acute rhinitis
common cold
acute tonsillitis

Respiratory system
acute bronchitis
asthma

Disorders of the eyes
acute conjunctivitis
central retinitis
myopia
cataract (without complications)

Disorders of the mouth
toothache
pain after tooth extraction
gingivitis
pharyngitis

Gastro-intestinal disorders
hiccoughs
gastritis
duodenal ulcers
colitis
constipation
diarrhoea

Neurological and musculo-skeletal disorders
headache
migraine
trigeminal neuralgia

General disorders
facial palsy
paralysis after a stroke
Menière's disease
nocturnal enuresis
frozen shoulder
tennis elbow
sciatica
low back pain
osteoarthritis

In addition a number of researchers have shown that acupuncture can be used to help relieve the pain of childbirth.

ALEXANDER TECHNIQUE

The background

The Alexander Technique was founded at the turn of the century by an Australian actor called F. Matthias Alexander who believed that many common illnesses are caused by our failure to use our bodies properly.

Alexander started his researches when he repeatedly lost his voice on stage. Doctors were unable to help him, patent medicine sprays helped his hoarseness only a little and more and more often he found himself losing his voice in mid performance. Desperate to find the cause he spent months standing in front of a mirror and attempting to work out why his voice kept disappearing.

Eventually, he found that when talking he had a habit of stiffening his neck and pulling his head backwards and downwards. This meant that his vocal cords got squashed and when he tried to correct the problem by deliberately putting his head forwards he again found himself pressing on his vocal cords. After months of work Alexander decided that the only solution was to change his posture and hold his body in such a way that his voice could be saved.

The Alexander 'technique' worked. Alexander found that once he had learned how to stand and hold his head his voice no longer kept on disappearing.

Alexander was so delighted by this discovery that he did not return to the stage. Instead he decided that since he had successfully managed to conquer his own problem by changing his posture then there was a good chance that other people would be able to benefit by changing their posture too. He created an educational programme aimed at eradicating bad posture and increasing self-awareness. The therapy (sometimes called The Alexander Technique and sometimes called The Alexander Principle) was designed to prevent illnesses developing and to treat problems which had already developed simply by training individuals to use their bodies gracefully, sensibly and according to their natural, mechanical strengths and weaknesses.

He, like so many others before him and after him, created a health philosophy out of personal experience.

To make a diagnosis

Teachers of the Alexander Technique are more interested in prevention than cure and more adept at eradicating bad habits than attacking existing symptoms directly.

The provision of treatment

Like osteopathy and chiropractic the Alexander Technique is based on the belief that the position of the bones, and the condition of the skeletal frame in general, can have a tremendous influence on the health of any individual.

F. M. Alexander believed that health can be restored and maintained simply by changing postural habits. He claimed that individuals who stand upright, with their backs straight and their heads held high, will have all their internal organs in exactly the right position. Such individuals would, he argued, be far less likely to develop any sort of disease or disorder. Alexander claimed that standing, walking and sitting properly would lead to a contented, comfortable and healthy lifestyle.

Today, teachers of the Alexander Technique follow Alexander's theories quite closely. They help patients to use their natural reflexes to stand and move comfortably and they help patients to use their bodies clearly, simply and effectively. They claim that by improving posture and movement it is also possible to improve breathing, digestion and circulation. One of their main aims is to help patients eradicate bad habits.

Although teachers of the Alexander Technique can certainly help their patients in many ways it is possible to take advantage of some of Alexander's research without taking formal lessons.

So, for example, begin by trying to visualize the way that you stand, sit and walk. If you have a friend with a video camera then persuade him or her to take a few shots of you in various positions. These shots will enable you to assess your movements critically, objectively and clinically. Examine the sort of things you do in a normal day. Do you always move, lift and carry things without putting an unnecessary strain on your body? Look at your shoes to see if there is any sign of uneven wear. Remember that uncomfortable shoes or sore feet can affect the way that you walk and end up producing serious joint and spine problems. Remember not to over-reach when picking up heavy objects and to lift heavy objects with your knees bent and your back straight.

Research

Apart from good anecdotes and enthusiastic testimonials from individuals (including orthodox physicians) who have tried the Alexander Technique, I know of no scientific evidence to show that Alexander's theories can do anything more than improve your posture and reduce your chances of developing joint, bone and muscle aches and pains.

Qualifications and training for the Alexander Technique

There are a number of colleges and training establishments where the Alexander Technique is taught. I know of no way to differentiate between the good, the bad and the grossly incompetent. I recommend, therefore, that readers follow the simple guidelines listed on page 22.

Dangers

There are few, if any, specific dangers associated with the Alexander Technique.

The uses of the Alexander Technique

The Alexander Technique is recommended for patients suffering from a wide range of disorders. Among those patients likely to benefit most are: patients suffering from mechanical (bone, joint and muscle) disorders; patients suffering from stress disorders; patients suffering from psychosomatic problems; patients convalescing after serious accidents, injuries or illnesses, and patients whose poor posture or bad habits have led to respiratory, digestive or circulatory problems.

ANTHROPOSOPHICAL MEDICINE

The background

Anthroposophical medicine is one aspect of a philosophy devised by Rudolf Steiner. Born in Austria in 1861 Steiner founded his basically spiritual movement on the notion that there is a spiritual world which can be reached by development of the perception beyond the physical senses to the level of pure thought. Steiner died in 1925.

Orthodox medicine is based on a purely physical world – on physical experiment and observation. Steiner believed that this attitude imposed unnecessary limits and claimed that thought, consciousness, perception and other experiences could also be useful. Anthroposophical medicine is not an alternative to but an extension of scientific medicine and is but one aspect of a much wider movement responsible for innovations in education, finance, agriculture and the arts.

The aim is to uncover the potential meaning and purpose of an illness while using treatments to promote healing. The doctor who follows anthroposophical medicine is encouraged to understand that there is more than a physical form to a human being.

Anthroposophical medicine is practised by doctors who have qualified in the conventional way.

To make a diagnosis

Doctors who practise anthroposophical medicine observe the patient's body in a conventional way but also look at the patient's personal history and examine his behaviour and history in a social context.

The provision of treatment

Anthroposophical practitioners use a wide variety of treatments. They may use homoeopathic doses of medicine or recommend special diets, massage or even art therapy.

Research

I know of no formal research work that validates anthroposophical medicine. But given the philosophical nature of anthroposophy it is difficult to see how any such research work could be done.

Qualifications and training for anthroposophical medicine

Anthroposophy is normally practised by doctors who have trained and qualified in the conventional way.

Dangers

I know of no specific dangers associated with this medical 'speciality'.

The uses of anthroposophy

Because of the wide range of treatment forms available to them there are no limitations to the diseases that can be treated by practitioners of this type.

APPLIED KINESIOLOGY

The background

The name 'applied kinesiology' was coined by Dr George J. Good-heart. The word 'kinesiology' means the science of movement and includes the anatomy, physiology and mechanics of muscle action.

Goodheart claimed that by examining and testing muscles and muscle movement he could identify major trouble spots in the bodies of his patients. Goodheart was a chiropractor and applied kinesiology was devised as an additional way of reaching a diagnosis.

To make a diagnosis

Chiropractors normally reach a diagnosis by examining the bones of their patients, by studying the way their patients move and stand, and by taking X-ray pictures. Applied kinesiology is merely another technique designed to enable chiropractors (and others) to identify offending vertebrae and find out exactly which joints need manipulating.

The provision of treatment

Applied kinesiology is designed to be used in conjunction with chiropractic.

Research

I know of no research evidence that proves the value of applied kinesiology.

Qualifications and training for applied kinesiology

As for chiropractic.

Dangers

Since this is a diagnostic tool which depends merely on observing and examining muscle movements there should not be any hazards associated with its use.

The uses of applied kinesiology

When Goodheart devised this technique he intended it to be used by chiropractors. However, these days, some practitioners claim that they can use applied kinesiology in all sorts of ways.

AROMATHERAPY

The background

Aromatherapists claim that by massaging their patients with sweet smelling oils they can treat an enormous range of physical and mental disorders. They say that by choosing scented oils from specific flowers, plants and trees they can influence moods and emotions and treat diseases.

Aromatherapy is a very traditional form of healing but the modern practice of aromatherapy seems to have been developed in Europe after the Second World War by Marguerite Maury and her husband.

To make a diagnosis

Different aromatherapists use different diagnostic techniques. Many seem to rely on intuition and conversation with their patients.

The provision of treatment

The aromatherapist concentrates on massaging the patient's back and face. A course of treatment may last for ten sessions.

Research

I know of no specific evidence to show that aromatherapy is of any real clinical value, but there is now a considerable amount of evidence to show that pleasant smells can have a quite remarkable effect. Back in 1938, for example, in a test conducted with a thousand women it was shown that when one pair of stockings out of four was faintly perfumed a total of 96 per cent of all the women tested thought that those stockings were the best of the bunch – even though all the stockings were, in fact, made of exactly the same material.

There is also evidence to show that olfactory influences are extremely effective at triggering off memories from the past. George Dodd and other research workers at Warwick University in England recently conducted some experiments with people under stress. They showed that when individuals were given stressful tasks to do, and at the same time exposed to an unfamiliar odour, they learned to associate the smell with the task. When they were later exposed to the smell alone they reacted to it as if they were under stress.

It is this sort of relationship between smells and experiences which explains why hospital smells strike fear into otherwise brave individuals and why some people drool over the smell of freshly mown grass or freshly spread tar.

In addition to there being evidence to show that particular perfumes can have a beneficial emotional effect, a relaxing massage with a pleasant smelling lubricant may be extremely beneficial.

Qualifications and training for aromatherapy

Most aromatherapists learn their skills from other aromatherapists – by a sort of apprenticeship. But it is possible to take a course in aromatherapy (part of it by correspondence).

Dangers

Apart from the risk of a patient being allergic to one of the oils used for massage I know of no specific hazards associated with aromatherapy.

The uses of aromatherapy

Aromatherapy is said to be good for skin problems, rheumatism, sinus troubles, poor circulation and depression. I have been unable to find any evidence at all to support any of these claims. It is, however, perfectly possible that a relaxing massage in pleasant surroundings with a good smelling lubricant may be beneficial (see also page 130).

ART THERAPY

The background

Art therapy – using painting as a therapeutic aid – is growing in popularity.

Those who advocate art therapy believe that painting helps patients express deep levels of thought, enables patients to free themselves from superficial restrictions and helps to provide an outlet for buried feelings and conflicts.

Art therapy has been practised in many different forms for centuries.

To make a diagnosis

Art therapists must either rely on their intuition or on diagnoses made by other practitioners.

The provision of treatment

Some art therapists work with orthodox medical practitioners – often in hospital units. Others work alone.

The patient is encouraged to use paints quite freely and without restraint.

Research

Some psychiatrists claim that art therapy can help patients but the evidence is anecdotal rather than scientific.

Qualifications and training for art therapy

No special qualifications or training are needed for art therapy, nor, as far as I know, are there any formal courses available in art therapy.

Dangers

I know of no specific dangers associated with art therapy although of course it is possible that a patient could be unbalanced by seeing what he or she had painted while suffering from depression or hallucinations.

The uses of art therapy

Art therapy is most often used to help patients with mental disorders.

AUTO-SUGGESTION

Emile Coue (1857–1926), a French chemist, is the father of auto-suggestion. After studying hypnotherapy Coue concluded that it is not the words or actions of the hypnotherapist that work so much as the stimulation of the patient's imagination.

The imagination is, he claimed, the key to self-help and self-treatment. Coue's basic message was that if a patient sows the idea that he is going to recover in his own mind then nature will take care of the rest.

Coue is remembered for the phrase 'Every day in every way I am getting better and better.'

To make a diagnosis

Auto-suggestion is a self-help treatment technique rather than a complete form of 'alternative' medicine. There are no specific diagnostic skills associated with auto-suggestion.

The provision of treatment

Auto-suggestion is widely practised under many different modern guises. (See also *Visualization*, page 177).

Research

No specific research has been done to prove the value of auto-suggestion but there is a considerable amount of anecdotal evidence available to show its worth.

Qualifications and training for auto-suggestion

There are no specific training programmes for auto-suggestion although similar philosophies are used by many active practitioners.

Dangers

I know of no specific dangers associated with auto-suggestion.

The uses of auto-suggestion

Auto-suggestion (in its many different forms) can be used to help patients fight and sometimes recover from all physical and most mental disorders.

AUTOGENIC TRAINING

The background

In the nineteenth century two scientists called Vogt and Brodmann of the Berlin Neuro-Biological Institute discovered that some of their patients were able to put themselves into semi-hypnotic states. They also discovered that this condition had a positive, healing effect. Patients who were able to calm and relax themselves were far less likely to need medical attention than patients who were continually feeling harassed and anxious.

In the 1930s a German psychiatrist rediscovered the work of Vogt and Brodmann. Impressed by it he decided to investigate the therapeutic possibilities of this type of self-hypnosis.

Eventually he called the approach 'autogenics' and it became known as 'autogenic training'.

To make a diagnosis

Autogenic training is a treatment programme designed to help patients who are suffering from symptoms produced by over-exposure to stress. Patients usually select themselves for autogenic training and there is no formal diagnostic regime associated with the technique.

The provision of treatment

Described by some observers as a Western version of yoga and transcendental meditation, autogenic training consists of six basic exercises. The patient repeats to himself the phrase which makes up each exercise until he is experiencing the suggested effect. Then he goes on to the next exercise.

The six phrases used by autogenic practitioners are (with some slight variations):

1   My arms and legs are heavy . . .
2   My arms and legs are warm . . .
3   My heart is calm and regular . . .
4   My breathing is calm and regular . . .
5   My abdomen is warm . . .
6   My forehead is cool . . .

Research

Autogenic training was devised by doctors who had an orthodox training and is often practised by doctors who have had an orthodox training. It is, therefore, not surprising that there is plenty of research evidence to show that autogenic training works. Over 2,500 scientific publications have proved that individuals who follow the autogenic exercises do benefit.

Qualifications and training for autogenic training

Autogenic training is usually practised by formally qualified medical practitioners.

Dangers

I know of no specific dangers associated with autogenic training.

The uses of autogenic training

Autogenic training is no better, and probably no worse, than any other form of relaxation therapy. The useful effects that are undoubtedly associated with its use are due not to the 'magic' of the incantations or to the skills of the practitioner involved but to the body's innate capacity for self-healing. It is the patient's own healing strengths which are responsible for any success associated with the remedy.

In my view autogenic training merely allows medical practitioners to introduce the interventionist philosophy into relaxation and self-healing.

The real advantage of self-healing techniques is that they can be used without professional support.

AYURVEDIC MEDICINE

The background

Ayurvedic medicine is a type of medicine that was founded in Asia and is commonly practised today by Asians. Ayurvedic practitioners are known as hakims or vaids.

The philosophy behind ayurvedic medicine is that it is possible to restore a patient to good health by balancing the forces coming from the individual with those of the environment. Practitioners examine the birthdate, age and pulse of the patient and balance that information with the climate and the positions of the stars.

To make a diagnosis

Ayurvedic practitioners use personal and environmental information in order to arrive at a diagnosis.

The provision of treatment

Hakims or vaids use up to a thousand different remedies. Sometimes they recommend that special foods be cooked for the patient. They do occasionally to use potentially dangerous heavy metals such as lead in the treatment of some conditions.

Research

I know of no formal or informal research evidence which proves the value of ayurvedic medicine.

Qualifications and training for ayurvedic medicine

This is a type of 'folk' medicine. Some training is available in India but I doubt if more than a small percentage of those practising this type of treatment have received any formal training.

Dangers

Some of the treatments used by ayurvedic practitioners are, in my view, potentially hazardous.

The uses of ayurvedic medicine

Practitioners claim that this type of treatment can be used for a wide range of physical and mental conditions. I know of no condition for which I would recommend any ayurvedic medicine.

BACH FLOWER REMEDIES

The background

Dr Edward Bach (1886–1936), a qualified doctor and homoeopath, believed that sickness and disease are a result of disharmony that exists deep within the patient, and claimed that this disharmony could be eased with the aid of simple, harmless remedies made from wild flowers.

To make a diagnosis

Being a homoeopath Bach believed that it was more important to treat the individual patient than to tackle the disease from which he was suffering. He prescribed his flower remedies according to the patient's psychological state and used his intuition to tell him what remedies to select.

The provision of treatment

To prepare the treatments flower heads are placed in water in a plain glass bowl and left in the sunlight. The water is then bottled to produce the flower-remedy medicine. To administer the remedy to a patient a couple of drops of this liquid are added to a glass of ordinary water.

Research

There is no research to show the value of flower remedies. Despite the fact that he had qualified as a doctor Edward Bach seems to have based his practice on intuition.

Qualifications and training for Bach flower remedies

All sorts of practitioners use the Bach remedies today. Most of the practitioners have no formal medical training of any kind.

Dangers

Bach seems to have been careful to make sure that none of his flower remedies was poisonous. The dilutions used mean that there are probably few hazards with this type of treatment.

The uses of Bach flower remedies

Edward Bach was undoubtedly a gentle, well-intentioned man, but it is difficult to see what possible value his remedies can have. He was, I suspect, a harmless nutter, and it seems surprising that people should still be making money out of his theories.

BATES EYESIGHT THERAPY

The background

In the first years of this century Dr W. D. Bates, an American eye specialist who practised in New York, did research work on eye diseases which led him to the conclusion that defective vision is not due to permanent changes in the shape of the eye but functional derangements.

Dr Bates argued that when the eye is used to look at an object, the external muscles which surround the eyeball are used to change the shape of the eye itself. He claimed that when a distant object is being examined, the external muscles move the back of the eye towards the lens, and that when a close object is being examined the opposite happens. He suggested that these muscular changes alter the shape of the eyeball and argued that individuals who are myopic (short-sighted) or hypermetropic (long-sighted) have eyeballs which have been misshapen by faulty action of the external muscles.

According to Bates, when a patient is myopic his eyeball is kept in a position which makes the viewing of distant objects difficult. On the other hand, when a patient suffers from hypermetropia the eyeball is kept in such a shape that the viewing of near objects is difficult.

So, Bates argued, if people with defective vision are really suffering because the external muscles of their eyeballs have been strained then they should be able to improve their vision by learning to relieve the strain and tension on their eye muscles.

When Bates put his theory into practice he found that it worked.

To make a diagnosis

The Bates techniques are recommended solely for the sort of eyesight problems that would normally be corrected by wearing spectacles.

The provision of treatment

Bates, writing some years before the Austrian endrocrinologist Hans Selye and his acolytes started to write about stress, suggested that many people with strained eye muscles suffer from mental tension which has set up a corresponding physical strain on the eyes and, in particular on the muscles which control them.

Bates believed that tense, nervous individuals are more likely to develop defective vision than others and he stated that overwork, worry, fear and anxiety can all help damage the eyesight.

Bates decided that the answer was to encourage his patients to learn how to relax themselves properly. He advocated both general exercises, designed to relax the whole body, and specific exercises, designed to relax the muscles around the eyeball.

The following regime, taken from my book *Bodypower*, is based on the Bates philosophies and on Harry Benjamin's book *Better Sight without Glasses*.

1   First, you must learn how to relax your body and your mind. You will find all the advice you need about how to relax on page 137.
2   If you have ever stared at something very hard you will know that the muscles of your eyes can get so tired that you eventually have to turn away and relax a little. Dr Bates had a technique called 'palming' which he recommended to patients who wanted to know how to relax their eyes effectively. To do this you should sit in a very comfortable position, as loose and as relaxed as you can get. Then close your eyes and cover them with your hands. Don't press on your eyes and leave your hands slightly cupped. There should be no direct pressure on your eyes at all.
    Now you either let the blackness gently fill your mind or, if you find it easier, allow images from your personal store of memories to fill your mind. (I suggest that you read the section on mental relaxation and daydreaming, page 137.) You should do this for ten minutes at a time, three times a day if you have defective vision. Otherwise, you should do it wherever your eyes feel tired.
3   You should exercise the muscles of your neck and shoulders. If these are tight they will have a bad effect on the small muscles around your eyes. First, raise your shoulders high. Then lower

them. Do this a few times, after which you should try pushing your shoulders back as far as possible. When you've done that a few times, move your head as far forward as you can – try to touch your chest with your chin. Then move your head back so that your chin is as far away from your chest as possible. Finally, try turning your head to the right as far as it will go and then to the left as far as it will go. These are exercises that you should try if you get tension headaches or aching eyes.

4   You can also do some specific exercises to help relax the muscles around your eyes. Allow your eyes to go up into your head as far as possible. Keep your head still and don't strain the muscles at all – just take your eyes as far as they will go naturally. Next, do a similar exercise, taking your eyes as far left as they will go and then as far right as they will go. Again, keep your head as still as you can and don't strain your eyes. Finally, try holding up your index finger (either hand will do) a few inches in front of your eyes. Look at the finger and then look at any object in the distance. Look backwards and forwards between your finger and the large object ten times. Rest for a moment or two and then repeat the exercise. If you have defective vision you should practise these exercises several times a day.

5   You can use your imagination to improve your vision. Look at any line of print in this book. Concentrate hard on one word in the middle of the line and then close your eyes and imagine that you can see the one word more clearly defined than the other words in the line. Open your eyes and look at the line again. Close your eyes and repeat the exercise. Keep doing this and when the whole word looks more clearly defined than the other words concentrate on smaller and smaller words – finally picking out individual letters for the exercise.

Research

I have been unable to find any formal research evidence to show that the Bates technique works. But there is a considerable amount of anecdotal evidence.

Qualifications and training for Bates eyesight therapists

The Bates technique is used by practitioners of many different kinds. Many of these practitioners have merely read books or papers written by Bates and probably know no more about the technique than is written here.

Dangers

There are no hazards that I know of with the Bates technique.

It is, however, interesting to note that Bates himself (and some of his successors) argued that by wearing spectacles people with bad eyes are merely making their eyesight worse and perpetuating their need for artificial aids.

Bates pointed out that spectacles do nothing at all to help any existing problem but are offered merely as an interventionist aid. They are intended to help an individual cope with a problem – not to help him overcome it.

The main danger is that by helping the patient who has defective vision to see with artificial aids the optician is ensuring that any muscle imbalance is maintained. The eyes are being prevented from recovering.

The uses of the Bates technique

By using the Bates technique some people who are prescribed spectacles can learn to manage without them – giving them up in easy stages.

If you wear spectacles and want to try without them, leave them off when you are relaxing, reading or messing around the home. Do the exercises I have described. Gradually you may find that you have to replace your spectacles with weaker lenses.

I do not think there is anything to be gained from visiting a Bates therapist.

BIOCHEMICS (BIOCHEMISTRY)

The background

The term 'biochemics' was coined by Dr William Schuessler (1821–98), a nineteenth-century homoeopath who worked in Germany and who claimed that there are, in the human body, twelve essential minerals (he called them tissue salts) which have vital and quite specific functions.

The tissue salts of Dr Schuessler include calcium phosphate, ferrous phosphate, calcium sulphate, potassium sulphate, sodium chloride, sodium sulphate, magnesium phosphate and calcium fluoride.

To make a diagnosis

Dr Schuessler (and those who follow his theory) claim that certain specific symptoms show that a patient is short of one or more tissue salts – for example, a lack of sodium will lead to digestive troubles and rheumatism.

The provision of treatment

Biochemics (which is also known, rather confusingly, as biochemistry) is based on a simple principle. When a tissue salt is missing then it is replaced by mouth. Biochemics is a purely physical remedy.

Research

I have been unable to find any research at all which substantiates the claims made by the late Dr Schuessler.

Qualifications and training for biochemics

The twelve tissue salts that are used in biochemics can be bought through the mail and patients are encouraged to treat themselves.

Dangers

I know of no specific dangers associated with this type of self-treatment.

The uses of biochemics

I cannot think of a single use for which I would recommend the so-called science of 'biochemics'.

BIOENERGETICS

The background

Austrian psychoanalyst Wilhelm Reich (1897–1957) believed that there is a universal energy source or life force called 'bioenergy' that is a vital ingredient to physical and mental health. Much of Reich's life was dedicated to helping people liberate this life force within their bodies and his followers still believe in the bioenergetics force.

To make a diagnosis

Bioenergetics is more a way of staying healthy than dealing with specific disease processes and so diagnostic skills are not important.

The provision of treatment

Reich believed that the mind and the body are interdependent. The practice of bioenergetics involves the release of tension and repressed emotions through massage and through special exercises. Reich also believed that sexual orgasm is a crucial safety valve designed to help liberate the mind and the body. He regarded each orgasm as a sign of proper functioning and free energy flow.

Research

I know of no formal research work which supports any of Reich's theories about bioenergetics.

Qualifications and training for bioenergetics

Some of Reich's followers have studied psychoanalysis (see

Psychotherapy, page 155). Others have merely read books written by or about him.

Dangers

I know of no specific hazards associated with bioenergetics. Although it is, of course, possible that the constant search for orgasmic release could lead to physical infection and emotional distress.

The uses of bioenergetics

Bioenergetics is of modest interest to medical historians.

BIOFEEDBACK

The background

Biofeedback practitioners use special, electrical machinery developed in the 1960s to help them monitor brain waves, heart beats, blood pressure, body temperature and other involuntary bodily functions. For obtaining information about brain-wave patterns they use an electroencephalograph (ECG). For measuring muscle tension they use an electromyograph (EMG). For measuring temperature they use a thermometer probe. And for measuring skin resistance they use an electrical skin resistance meter.

By attaching patients to the right sort of equipment, biofeedback practitioners can monitor changes in body physiology. It is then possible to use those variations to help patients cope with their own headaches, heart problems, high blood pressure, circulatory disorders and so on. The biofeedback machines translate subtle changes into auditory or visual signals. And by listening to and watching these changes the patient is able to see how his body is changing and responding to different circumstances.

When biofeedback first became popular early in the 1970s it was forecast that people would eventually be able to control all phobias and anxieties, that there would be a fall in the use of drugs and hospitals, that psychiatrists would all be put out of business and that patients would be able to deal with many threatening disorders themselves.

One biofeedback practitioner forecast that biofeedback machinery would eventually enable employers to select the right people for high-pressure jobs and would enable men and women to find their perfect marriage partners. Another expert said that men would be able to control their own fertility by changing their scrotal temperature.

To make a diagnosis

Biofeedback machinery does nothing more than identify specific physiological changes. There are no diagnostic skills associated with biofeedback.

The provision of treatment

Biofeedback has some value as a research tool, but for two main reasons its practical applications are limited.

The first problem is that biofeedback systems are designed to measure specific aspects of body activity. One system is needed to measure the pulse, another to measure temperature and a third to measure blood pressure. The equipment is expensive, fairly cumbersome and, often, difficult to use. Much of the equipment can only be used in the laboratory.

The second problem is that biofeedback systems tend to be 'disease-specific'. A patient who has learned to use biofeedback to help her cope with her high blood pressure won't be able to use what she has learned to help her deal with her migraine attacks.

Research

Countless research papers have been published to show the technical value of biofeedback.

Qualifications and training for biofeedback

Biofeedback machinery can be demonstrated by anyone who has a little training.

Dangers

I know of no particular hazards which are associated with the use of biofeedback.

The uses of biofeedback

When biofeedback was first introduced it seemed to have a great future. The idea behind it was very simple. A patient with, for example, high blood pressure would be wired up to a biofeedback machine showing a blood-pressure reading. The patient would then be encouraged to relax his mind. As the patient relaxed so he would see his blood pressure fall.

It was thought that by showing an immediate relationship between high blood pressure and relaxation it would be possible to teach patients how to control their own disorders quickly, easily and safely.

In practice this has not happened. Biofeedback has turned out to be of more value in the research laboratory than in the consulting room. Patients can benefit from relaxation exercises (and so on) without using biofeedback machinery.

BIOMAGNETIC THERAPY

For forty years or more scientists have argued that the human body produces a powerful magnetic field and that this internal magnetic field can be influenced and damaged by electro-magnetic radiation from outside the body. There are, inevitably perhaps, also manufacturers who claim that they can sell machines which stimulate or regulate the body's own magnetic field. The phrase 'biomagnetic therapy' is sometimes used to describe these machines.

To make a diagnosis

Sophisticated equipment is available which is said to enable practitioners to measure the body's electro-magnetic pulsations.

The provision of treatment

Equally sophisticated (and impressive-looking) equipment is available which is said to enable practitioners to treat electro-magnetic disorders.

Research

I know of no independent research work which proves the practical, clinical value of biomagnetic therapy.

Qualifications and training for biomagnetic therapy

I am unaware of any special training or qualifications for biomagnetic therapy.

Dangers

I do not know what dangers there may be associated with biomagnetic therapy. I suspect that I am not alone in my ignorance.

The uses of biomagnetic therapy

I have seen biomagnetic therapy recommended for: migraine, headache, tension, depression, tiredness, nervousness, psychosomatic disorders, nervous stomach, sleeplessness, loss of vitality, loss of concentration, travel sickness, jet lag and pain.

My own view is that biomagnetic therapy is of no value whatsoever.

BIORHYTHMS

The background

Our lives are greatly influenced by rhythms of one sort or another. The spinning of the Earth around its central axis gives us our days and our nights and provides us with a pattern for living. We sleep and work, rest and play, eat and drink according to the daily rhythm which results from the Earth's continual movement.

But that is just one of the many rhythms which have an effect on the way we live. There is, for example, the rhythm that ensures that a woman's hormone levels will rise and fall in such a way that she will alternately ovulate and menstruate, allowing each fresh egg to have its chance, then seeing that it is discarded at the right moment. There is an internal clock which controls body temperature from day to day and which, for some reason which no one yet entirely understands, seems to match the menstrual cycle.

There is much more that we don't yet understand about body rhythms. We don't know why blood pressure varies from day to day. Or why the best time to learn something is just before we go to sleep. Or why the best time for making important decisions is in the middle of the day. Or why most of us are alert during the early evening. Or why more people die at 4.00 am than at any other time of day or night.

There are body clocks which govern what takes place when we fall asleep. There is evidence to show that epileptics always tend to have their fits at much the same sort of time of day. And there is research which shows that there is a link between depression and some sort of body rhythm.

And, of course, there is the undeniable fact that we all seem to have some good days and some bad days.

With all this information available it is hardly surprising that some observers now argue that there is a fundamental rhythm which governs all aspects of life. A rhythm that offers a single explanation for our swings in skill, mood and capacity.

The theory of biorhythms was first put forward by two scientists who arrived at much the same conclusion at the beginning of the century. In Berlin an otorhinolaryngologist called Wilhelm Fleiss (1858–1928) was trying to explain why there should be such a wide variation in the interval between individuals being exposed to disease and the emergence of clinical signs and symptoms. In Vienna, Hermann Swoboda, a professor of psychology, was struggling with a discovery that dreams, ideas, fears, worries and creative urges all occur in patterns which seem to fit birth dates.

The two scientists arrived at similar conclusions quite separately; announcing within a couple of years of one another that our physical vitality and strength is governed by a 23-day cycle while our emotional strength and stability is governed by a 28-day cycle. A few years later a third scientist, Professor Alfred Teltscher of Innsbruck, declared that there is a third, 33-day cycle, which governs intellectual activity.

All three cycles are said to begin on our birthdays and to follow a wave pattern after that – with the three waves repeating themselves after 23, 28 and 33 days. The theory is that the peaks and troughs of each cycle are the most critical times and that on those days an individual is particularly likely to be at his best or at his worst.

Fairly recently, Professor K. Tatai, head of behavioural sciences at Tokyo University, mixed the three cycles together to create the combined reading that many people know as a complete biorhythm.

To make a diagnosis

Biorhythms are a fortune-telling aid. By a careful study of the way that the three waves relate to one another, it is, theoretically at least, possible to select the most suitable times of the month for particular types of action.

It is alleged that if the date of a surgical operation is picked with care then the patient's chances of making a good recovery will be much enhanced.

The provision of treatment

There is no treatment associated with biorhythms.

Research

Many attempts have been made to find genuine evidence of links between biorhythms and accidents or illnesses. But so far no one has managed to find any convincing evidence at all. For example, a study undertaken by the British Transport and Road Research Laboratory into the biorhythms of drivers involved in road traffic accidents showed no significant correlation at all.

Qualifications and training for biorhythms

Books, charts and computer software are available for those who want to learn how to use biorhythms.

Dangers

I know of no specific dangers associated with biorhythms.

The uses of biorhythms

People have always rather liked the idea of there being some great unexplained influence on their lives. And now that religion is on the wane and astrology, although extremely popular, is regarded with some suspicion there are many who find the idea of biorhythms extremely attractive.

Biorhythms do, after all, offer a seemingly logical and scientifically acceptable answer to the fact that we all have an apparently unpredictable mixture of good and bad days.

But the fact is that there is no real evidence to prove that biorhythms are of any genuine value. They should be regarded as being in the same general category as forecasts made by newspaper astrologers.

CELL REVITALIZATION THERAPY

The background

Cell therapy was first made famous by Paul Neihans of Switzerland. The aim is to revitalize the body by introducing brand new cells. According to one advertisement cell replacement therapy is 'a kind of transplant, by means of intra-muscular injections, of cellular material containing the active elements of the cell'.

A good many elderly politicians and show-business personalities have spent money on cell therapy. Among the better known names are: Winston Churchill, Charles de Gaulle, Konrad Adenauer, Dwight Eisenhower, the Duke of Windsor, Cary Grant, Charles Chaplin, Marlene Dietrich, Gloria Swanson and Somerset Maugham.

The cells that are injected into the patient usually come from lambs.

To make a diagnosis

Practitioners talk to their patients to find out what symptoms are causing most concern. They also do tests to assess the levels of various hormones in the body.

The provision of treatment

Injections are usually given twice a week for up to a month.

Research

I know of absolutely no research to show that cell replacement therapy is of any value at all.

Qualifications and training for cell revitalization therapy

Those who practise this type of treatment usually appear to have impressive qualifications, but it is sometimes difficult to assess the real value of those qualifications.

Dangers

There may or may not be serious risks associated with cell revitalization therapy.

The uses of cell revitalization therapy

CRT practitioners claim that it will treat conditions such as: poor general physical and mental ability, poor memory and concentration, convalescence following illness, poor skin tone and muscle tone, dry and greasy skin, menstrual cycle problems, premenstrual tension, fluid retention, headaches, backache, excessive perspiration, night cramps, difficulty in passing water, hormonal imbalance, digestive problems, insomnia. It is also said to be good for sexual problems.

When asked, 'What can the treatment really do for me?' one practitioner replies, 'It depends on what is wrong with you.'

Personally, I firmly believe that this type of cell therapy has, at best, a placebo effect. In my view these practitioners take advantage of the Gafes, fears and anxieties of those who are elderly, frail or inadequate. They represent, I believe, the completely unacceptable face of alternative medicine.

CHIROPRACTIC

The background

Chiropractic – the twentieth-century equivalent of bonesetting – was established in the last few years of the nineteenth century by a Canadian named Daniel David Palmer.

Palmer believed that 95 per cent of all illnesses were caused by displaced vertebrae (the technical term he used for displacement was 'subluxation') and after managing to restore the hearing of a janitor who had been deaf for seventeen years Palmer was convinced that the spine was the key to good health and that spinal manipulations would deal with most if not all illnesses.

Because of Palmer's rather extreme views, and obviously outrageous claims, chiropractic was, from the start, opposed by the medical establishment.

Chiropractors still believe that when parts of the body's bony frame are displaced they can press against nerves – causing pain and many other symptoms. Some chiropractors believe that by manipulating bones and joints they can not only help deal with specific structural problems but also help relieve internal problems involving non-bony organs such as the heart and lungs.

It is, however, only fair to point out that today many chiropractors do hold far less extreme views, recognizing that chiropractic cannot deal with every ailment.

To make a diagnosis

Traditionally chiropractors use their hands to help them reach a diagnosis. But they also talk to their patients and many modern chiropractors use X-rays to help them reach specific diseases.

The provision of treatment

Treatment from a chiropractor usually involves manipulation. The most important items of equipment that a chiropractor uses are his hands, although it is common for chiropractors to use a specially built couch so that their manipulations can be particularly effective.

Although chiropractic is still primarily concerned with the spine, practitioners also offer exercise regimes, dietary advice and all sorts of non-specific counselling. Moreover most modern practitioners do recognize that chiropractic cannot deal with every ailment.

Research

Although chiropractic is a long-established medical 'alternative' I have been unable to find independent research evidence to show the value of this speciality.

Qualifications and training for chiropractic

There are numerous colleges and societies around the world for chiropractors. There is no reliable way of assessing the value of a chiropractor's academic qualifications.

Dangers

Chiropractic manipulation of the spine can be dangerous if it is done carelessly or without the proper investigations. (See also *Osteopathy*, page 147.)

The uses of chiropractic

Although some chiropractors still claim that chiropractic can be used to treat almost any disease it seems clear that chiropractic is particularly useful for disorders of the bones and joints.

It is, for example, helpful in the treatment of backache, headaches, hip problems, and many other joint disorders. It is also good for neck, shoulder and arm pains. Chiropractic is not, however, a sensible form of treatment for cancer, gout, generalized rheumatism, osteoarthritis of the hips or fractured bones.

CHRISTIAN SCIENCE

The background
Christian Scientists believe that to conquer illness one must only accept the importance of God's power. Mary Baker Eddy, the American-born founder of this movement, preached that the key influence in health and healing was the state of the patient's mind. Mary Baker Eddy insisted that Christian Scientists should have nothing at all to do with doctors but should 'think' themselves well.

To make a diagnosis
Christian Scientists don't bother with diagnoses.

The provision of treatment
Treatment is in God's hands.

Research
There is none.

Qualifications and training for Christian Science
There is but one practitioner and as far as I know He has had no formal training.

Dangers
There are no specific dangers associated with Christian Science although there is a very considerable risk that patients will delay too long before seeking orthodox medical help.

The uses of Christian Science
Since 90 per cent of all illnesses are self-healing it is clear that Christian Scientists can expect a good success rate.

CLINICAL ECOLOGY

The background

Clinical ecologists believe that a wide range of diseases and symptoms (including physical disorders as varied as indigestion, palpitations, and headaches, and mental disorders such as depression) are caused by allergies to foods or other substances such as pesticides, inorganic fertilizers and pollutants.

To make a diagnosis

In order to find out what is causing an allergy reaction clinical ecologists will usually insist that the patient be isolated from all possible allergens. The symptoms should then clear up and reappear when the offending allergen is reintroduced.

The provision of treatment

In most cases treatment involves avoiding the cause of the allergy reaction.

Research

There is a considerable amount of anecdotal evidence (but remarkably little scientific evidence) to show that diseases are caused by allergens and that symptoms can be conquered by controlling the patient's exposure to those allergens.

Qualifications and training for clinical ecologists

Some clinical ecologists are registered medical practitioners who have had a normal, formal medical training. Others have had very little formal training of any kind.

Dangers

There are few, if any, specific hazards associated with clinical ecology.

The uses of clinical ecology

Patients who suspect that their symptoms could be caused by an allergy to a specific substance may gain considerably from a consultation with a clinical ecologist.

COLOUR THERAPY

The background

There is now a growing amount of evidence to suggest that we are all affected by colours and that the colours we choose tell others a good deal about the way we think and act. Some psychologists are now so confident that colour coding people pays off that they use colour tests to help employers recruit new members of staff. Experts such as Max Luscher believe that it is possible to assess personality very accurately by checking a whole series of colour preferences.

To make a diagnosis

Some experts hand patients a whole series of coloured cards and ask them to put the cards in order of preference. The sequence of colours chosen is particularly important. So, for example, some experts believe that an individual who picks grey and then red is probably not very trustworthy.

Other colour experts study the colour of an individual's clothes and even the colour of the ink in his or her pen. Use red ink and you'll be branded as pig-headed. Use violet ink and the psychologist will put you down as 'dominating'.

The provision of treatment

Many researchers around the world have shown that specific colours will help particular patients. So, for example, researchers at the University of California have claimed that yellow helps people lose weight, green helps convalescent patients, violet helps depression while turquoise is good for spots.

A psychologist from Boston University has suggested that a patient who has difficulty in getting to sleep or relaxing should trying gazing at something blue for twenty minutes or so. Blue is, it is said, a calming colour which relieves tension and reduces the blood pressure.

Researchers at Cambridge University have found that red light lowers the pain threshold (and puts up the heart rate).

Research

Researchers have spent a great deal of time investigating the value of colour. Not all their research has been valuable. When the director of biosocial research at City College in Tacoma, Washington claimed that the colour pink could turn aggressive individuals into calm, quiet, reasonable souls a prison governor in San Jose, California had his cells painted pink to try out the theory. He found that it worked for about fifteen minutes. After twenty minutes the men got over their shock and their innate aggressiveness began to return. Prisoners who were left in their pink cells for more than three hours started to tear the paint off the walls. The prison governor concluded that pink is great for cells where the inmates have sentences of no more than fifteen minutes.

Qualifications and training for colour therapy

Most colour therapists are psychologists.

Dangers

I know of no specific hazards associated with colour therapy.

The uses of colour therapy

Drug companies have been using colours therapeutically for years. They believe that blue is the best colour for heart drugs, yellow is best for anxiety, green is the best colour for tranquillizers, orange for stimulating the appetite and red for pain. These associations seem to be fairly universal but there are some colour associations which are national and drug companies which sell drugs around the world have to be careful. For example, the company which tried to promote a blue contraceptive pill in a blue package to Indian women had a real problem. The Indian ladies regarded blue as a colour for women with a rather less than immaculate moral character.

Hospital designers have had their difficulties too. The colour recommended for recovery rooms and intensive care units is purple. I know of one hospital where the intensive care unit had to be repainted when it was discovered that the purplish walls were making all the patients look cyanosed and close to death.

Colour therapy has its uses but it can produce plenty of problems too.

CUPPING

The background

Cupping is an ancient technique used to draw blood to the surface of the skin.

To make a diagnosis

Cupping is a form of treatment.

The provision of treatment

A tumbler or thick glass cup is first heated and then placed on the skin. Alternatively a small flame is placed inside a container to burn up oxygen and create a vacuum. A third method of treatment is to create a vacuum by sucking air out of the glass with a rubber tube. Whatever technique is used the vacuum ensures that the skin underneath becomes red and unusually well supplied with blood.

Research

There is no research that I know of to show the value of cupping.

Qualifications and training for cupping

No qualifications are required and little training is needed for cupping.

Dangers

The skin can be damaged.

The uses of cupping

Cupping was once used in the treatment of rheumatism and other joint disorders. It has also been used for chest problems such as asthma. I can think of no condition for which I would today recommend cupping.

DANCE THERAPY

The background

Dance therapy has been used for centuries. It is today used to teach patients better coordination and self-awareness. However, in addition to the physical benefits there are also said to be psychological and emotional benefits.

To make a diagnosis

Dance therapy does not involve the making of a diagnosis.

The provision of treatment

Patients can benefit from just about any kind of rhythmic dance therapy. The most important thing is that the patient should enjoy the accompanying music and find it easy to dance to. Those criteria are far more important than whether the music is classical or modern.

Research

There is a growing amount of anecdotal evidence to show that dance therapy is of value with some patients – particularly those who are mentally retarded or physically handicapped in some way.

Qualifications and training for dance therapy

Dance therapy is usually taught by trained dancers.

Dangers

There are, to my knowledge, no specific hazards associated with dance therapy. Although it is, of course, true that over-enthusiasm can lead to muscle sprains and strains.

The uses of dance therapy

Dance therapy is an excellent way of restoring function to stiffened or damaged muscles or joints. It is also an excellent way to banish loneliness and encourage acceptable social behaviour.

ENCOUNTER THERAPY

The background

Encounter therapy began in the 1940s when American psychologists began to experiment with different ways of developing and exploring human relationships. Working on the thesis that normal meetings between people are governed by an enormous number of social rules and restrictive conventions the encounter therapists tried to remove all normal barriers and encourage their patients to be totally uninhibited.

Individual patients are encouraged to abandon their prejudices and anxieties and to let themselves go, physically, verbally and emotionally. Every member of the group of patients involved is told to open up his or her deepest feelings and to share his fears, hopes and personal ambitions with other members of the group.

To make a diagnosis

Encounter therapy does not involve the making of a diagnosis.

The provision of treatment

Members of an encounter group are usually told to start by closing their eyes, walking around the room and exploring one another's bodies. They are then encouraged to express their own feelings in a way that is normally not considered acceptable among strangers. Encounter therapy sessions can often produce traumas and crises and patients are encouraged to get rid of their aggressions by screaming and shouting – as well as by assaulting cushions.

Research

Many psychologists have written about encounter therapy but I have been unable to find any independent evidence to show that encounter therapy is of any real, lasting value.

Qualifications and training for encounter therapy

Encounter therapy groups are sometimes organized by properly qualified psychologists and psychiatrists (a psychologist is someone who has studied the human mind, a psychiatrist is a medically qualified doctor who has studied disorders and diseases of the mind). But encounter therapy is often organized by individuals who have no formal training in either discipline.

Dangers

'Playing around' with the human mind can be very dangerous and encounter therapy is no exception. Patients who have hidden long established problems or who have forgotten and repressed former traumas can suffer badly during encounter therapy. There is a real risk that a mild, superficial anxiety can be turned into something far more devastating.

The uses of encounter therapy

The dangers of encounter therapy mean that it is probably not suitable for use outside some sort of mental health care institution. However, a version of encounter therapy is now widely used to help business executives improve their understanding of how people think and respond to crises. These sessions are probably harmless enough.

FASTING

The background

Fasting has been a popular type of treatment for centuries. Many of the great 'doctors' of the past – including Hippocrates, Galen and Paracelsus – have at one time or another recommended fasting as a way of purging the body. Plato claimed that fasting enabled him to think more clearly.

Today naturopaths (see page 144) believe that fasting helps to purge the body of waste materials and helps to detoxify it too. In addition there are numerous practitioners who recommend periods of fasting to patients who want to lose weight.

To make a diagnosis

There are no diagnostic skills associated with fasting.

The provision of treatment

Few things are easier to practise than fasting: you simply stop eating. In its purest form fasting means the complete absence of food and drink. In some cases, however, patients who are fasting are allowed to drink water or fruit juice.

Research

I know of no reliable research to show that fasting is a useful and safe form of treatment.

Qualifications and training for fasting

Fasting is recommended by a wide range of therapists – most of whom have no formal training.

Dangers

Side effects and unpleasant symptoms are common with fasting. Patients usually complain of headaches, vomiting and other side effects within a few hours of starting to fast. Other varied and often far more serious problems may ensue if the fast is persisted with. Those who recommend fasting claim that these symptoms are a sign that the body is getting rid of toxins and purifying itself. I know of no evidence to support these claims. It is, however, an undeniable fact that persistent fasting (particularly when fluids are avoided too) can be extremely dangerous and may lead to death.

The uses of fasting

There is none other than as the short-term (24–48 hours) treatment of food poisoning and similar problems.

HAIR ANALYSIS

The background

For many years now forensic laboratories have routinely used hair snippings to help them measure quantities of arsenic in the human body. The technique is normally used in murder cases when the police want to find out whether or not the grieving widow had been slipping her late lamented husband a little something extra in his porridge.

Not long ago a scientist found traces of arsenic in Napoleon Bonaparte's hair and there was quite a flurry among historians who thought that this might prove that Napoleon had been poisoned. Then scientists and historians alike realized that Napoleon had almost certainly been taking an arsenic-rich proprietary medicine for a stomach complaint that had plagued him for many years.

The chemicals which can be identified in hair snippings can be very revealing and forensic scientists can use a few locks of hair to help them identify individuals. Hair samples can be just as revealing and just as significant as fingerprints.

In the last few years a number of commercial laboratories have taken advantage of the principles of hair analysis and started to offer patients diagnoses and treatments based on single hair clippings sent in through the mail.

The patient simply chops off a couple of unwanted locks, pops them into an envelope and waits for the reply.

When the reply comes back, a few days later, it will usually suggest that the patient needs one or two vitamin and mineral supplements to restore his good health.

You may or may not be surprised to learn that the companies

providing the hair analysis service can usually sell you a supply of all the vitamins and minerals that they think you need.

To make a diagnosis

You send the laboratory a snipping of hair. The laboratory then uses a machine to identify some of the chemicals that are present in the hair. Based on this slender evidence the hair analyst will then recommend vitamin and mineral supplements that he thinks are necessary. Hair analysis is essentially a diagnostic service.

The provision of treatment

The treatment associated with hair analysis usually consists of vitamins and minerals. These are usually sold through the post. The prices may be very high. For more information about vitamin and mineral supplementation see page 182.

Research

Although hair analysis is a useful forensic tool I know of no evidence to suggest that hair analysis is a reliable way of making a medical diagnosis.

Qualifications and training for hair analysis

Forensic scientists are highly trained specialists. I have no reason to suspect that the individuals offering hair analysis services are either highly trained or specialists.

Dangers

Vitamin and mineral supplements can under some circumstances be dangerous. (See page 183.)

The uses of hair analysis

Hair analysis is, in my view , one of the worst examples of pseudo-science. But hair analysis still seems to thrive. The real weakness with this so-called science is that contact with water, dyes, hair restorers, shampoos and conditioners can all distort the readings that are obtained – as can the length of the hair and the site from which the sample was taken. Hair analysis is, to say the very least, an inexact science.

HEALING

The background

Healing has a remarkably long tradition – reaching far back beyond the origins of Christianity.

Some healers describe themselves as 'spiritual' and believe that their healing power comes directly from a god or superior being of some kind. Other healers say that they are merely a channel through which natural healing powers can succeed.

The difference between 'healing', 'spiritual healing' and 'faith healing' causes a considerable amount of confusion among both practitioners and patients. The fact is that there is a considerable amount of overlap between the different types of healing. These, however, are the definitions that are widely accepted:

Faith healing   The patient trusts the healer and allows his will-power and energies to be marshalled in such a way that he can make best use of his body's self-healing capacities. The patient must trust the healer and there is a powerful link between the patient's mind and his body.

Spiritual healing   The patient may or may not know that the healing is taking place. He may or may not be receptive and enthusiastic. The healer transmits energy from himself to the patient in some mysterious way.

Healing   The word is used very generally to describe the whole phenomenon.

In many instances when healing takes place the patient will be required to believe in some strong, supernatural force, some god or some religious being, who will offer a cure – usually in return for some form of prayer, supplication or pilgrimage.

One of the famous places where healing takes place is Lourdes, a town in the French Pyrenees which is worth discussing in some detail.

The history of Lourdes as an attraction for pilgrims seeking cures goes back to 1858 when a 14-year-old girl called Bernadette Soubiros claimed that a lady had appeared to her on the cliffs of Massabielle, a spot just outside Lourdes itself. The young girl's report of her conversation with this mysterious lady led the people of the town to believe that the lady she had met had been none other than the Blessed Virgin Mary – the Mother of Jesus Christ.

As a result Lourdes quickly became a favourite place of pilgrimage. Catholics from all over Europe wanted to visit the spot where the Virgin Mary had been seen. Among the pilgrims were a great many sick people hoping to be cured.

At first the local authorities weren't all that keen on the idea. They wanted to play the whole thing down. But local businessmen who were busy catering to the thousands of hungry and thirsty pilgrims were more enthusiastic. Within a short time the local bishop had decided that young Bernadette really had met the Virgin Mary. Lourdes had become an official place of pilgrimage.

In 1883 the Baron de St Maclou, a doctor, took up residence at Lourdes and started examining those people who claimed that they had been cured. He insisted on seeing medical certificates from patients who claimed that they had been healed and he invited all visiting members of the medical profession to take part in his investigations. Neither he nor the Catholic Church were particularly keen to have an epidemic of so-called miracles.

The system that the Baron devised is still followed today, over a century later. Everyone who claims to have been cured by a miracle at Lourdes must go before the Lourdes Medical Bureau which examines each individual very carefully. All the doctors attending Lourdes on any one day (and that can be over one hundred) are allowed to take part in the preliminary questioning of the patient who claims to have been cured by a miracle.

The Medical Bureau uses a set of simple rules (based on rules set up in 1735 by Cardinal Lambertini who later became Pope Benedict 14th) to help decide whether or not a miracle has taken place.

First, the disease that has been cured must be serious, normally incurable, and unlikely to have responded to treatment.

Second, a disease which disappears must not have reached a stage where it could have disappeared by itself.

Third, no medication should have been given to the patient. Or, if medicines were prescribed, then they must have had quite unimportant effects.

Fourth, the cure must be sudden and reached more or less instantaneously.

Finally, the cure must be complete.

If the Bureau decides that there is a possibility of a medically inexplicable cure then they open a dossier on the patient and invite him or her to return to Lourdes the following year. Meanwhile, the President of the Medical Bureau tries to collect as much information about the pilgrim as he possibly can.

For at least three years the pilgrim must return to Lourdes and be re-examined. Then, and only then, will the case be referred to the International Medical Committee of Lourdes. If *they* are convinced that the cure has no medical explanation then the Church will be invited to declare the healing a miracle.

Not surprisingly this doesn't happen very often. Over four million pilgrims go to Lourdes every year and about 65,000 are registered as sick. Since 1858 a total of 6,000 people claiming to have been cured miraculously have been examined. Of them only 64 have been recognized as official miracles.

As medical science advances and the Lourdes scrutineers find it more and more possible to explain seemingly inexplicable cures the number of miracles seems to decrease.

Lourdes is, of course, a unique centre for pilgrims looking for a miracle. Patients going there have tremendous faith in the generosity and kindness of their God.

Despite the popularity of places like Lourdes most healers claim that healing isn't necessarily mystical and certainly doesn't need to be associated with any religion or religious group.

The majority of healers claim that whereas the world 'faith' implies that healing must always come from some sort of religious power or divine intervention, their experience suggests that there is absolutely no need for an individual to have any faith. On the contrary they claim that healing is a natural phenomenon that all of us can benefit from.

'Healing,' one healer has said, 'is not a special gift. It is just that the full-time healers practise a lot and get quite good at it.'

Today healing (in all its varied forms) has become a thriving alternative medical speciality. There are tens of thousands of healers around. In Britain, for example, the Confederation of Healing Organizations represents no less than nine separate healing groups and some nine thousand individual healers.

To make a diagnosis

Healing is a therapy and there are not usually any diagnostic skills associated with it or its practitioners.

The provision of treatment

Healers work in a wide variety of different ways. Some healers lay their hands on their patients. Some put their hands just above the patient's body. Some healers claim that they can heal a patient without the patient being present (this is, not surprisingly, known as 'absent healing'). Some healers pray, some mutter incantations and some remain completely silent. Some encourage their patients to visualize (see *Visualization*, page 177) an improvement in their bodies. Some healers claim that they act on behalf of special healing forces.

Some healers charge their patients a fee. Some do not.

One thing that most healers agree on is that *anyone* can become a healer. Mothers can heal their children, orthodox doctors can heal their patients and we can all heal ourselves – some of the time at least.

The advantage of visiting a professional healer is that you benefit from that individual's strength of personality and enthusiasm. The good healer can give even the most cynical and timid patient vigour, energy and strength.

Loving someone, and wanting them to get better, are, it seems, part of the healing force. But there is more to it than that. The effective healer must want to help his patients but he must also be prepared to transfer some of his own healing energies to the minds and bodies of his patients.

Research

Like most other responsible practitioners healers are keen to obtain real evidence to show that they can help patients get better. And a number of experiments have already been conducted.

One of the earliest pieces of important research work was done by a biochemist called Bernard Grad who worked at McGill University in Montreal in the late 1950s and early 1960s. The subjects of his experiments were mice and plants.

In the first experiment the mice were operated on – each having a small patch of skin removed. The mice were then divided into two groups. The mice in the first group were touched by a healer. The mice in the second group were left to heal by themselves without any treatment at all. The experiment showed that when a healer touched the mice they got better much quicker than when they were left to get better alone. It was even shown that if the healer touched a mouse's bedding it would improve the speed with which he got better.

In the second experiment similarly impressive results were obtained with plants. Barley seeds were made 'sick' by putting them into a saline solution. Once again it was shown that the seeds which were touched by a healer made a much speedier recovery than the seeds which were not touched by a healer.

In America, Dolores Krieger, Professor of Nursing at New York University and one of the best known healers in the world, has convinced sceptical doctors by running controlled trials in which it has been shown that blood changes produced by healing can be measured in the laboratory. You can't get evidence much more conclusive than that.

I have for a long time been convinced that healers can produce a positive effect when dealing with patients (I suspect that healing stimulates the production of the body's own self-healing hormones) but I remained sceptical about the ability of healers to produce genuine physical changes until I made a series of programmes for BBC television.

Just before starting the series I had received a letter from a lady who practises healing and I had invited her to take part in one of the programmes. The healer had written to me claiming to have quite unusual healing powers and I wanted to check her out.

At my request the healer brought with her to the studio a patient who had suffered from bad arthritis and who claimed that her pains had 'miraculously' disappeared. My scepticism faded completely when I obtained the patient's X-rays from her hospital consultant and found that there had been an observed radiological improvement in the patient's condition.

Nor was this merely the result of my interpretation of the X-rays. We obtained reports written by an expert radiologist who didn't even know that the patient had seen a healer. His reports suggested that there had been a definite and otherwise inexplicable change in the patient's condition in the time when she had been seen by the healer.

Of course, a single patient's experiences – even supported by X-ray evidence – is not scientific proof. Much more evidence is needed before healing will be widely accepted by the medical profession. But there is now real hope that such evidence will soon be available.

Britain's Confederation of Healing Organizations has now devised a research project designed to evaluate the effect of healing on patients. Trials are currently under way with patients suffering from a variety of specific physical conditions – ranging from rheumatoid arthritis to cataracts.

Hopefully these experiments will provide evidence to show exactly what effect healing does have on illness and disease.

Meanwhile, there is a simple experiment that can be done by anyone who wants to be convinced of the possible 'healing power' of the human hands.

Start by putting your hands close together, with your fingers pointed away from you as though you were praying. Don't quite let your hands touch but get them as close together as you possibly can.

Now, separate your hands by about 2 inches and keep them apart for a few seconds.

Then return your hands to their original position – with the palms as close together as you can get them without touching.

Keep your hands in that position for a few seconds and then separate them by 4 inches. Once again keep them apart for a few seconds.

After returning your hands back to their original position separate them by 6 in. Do this as slowly as you possibly can and remember to stay in each different position for a few seconds at a time.

Finally, separate your hands by 8 or 10 inches and then slowly bring them back together again in rather jerky, 2 inch movements.

You will quite possibly feel a strange sort of 'bounciness', as though air were being compressed between your hands. And you'll probably also notice a change in the skin temperature of your hands. It may become a little warmer or simply tingle a little, but with most people the changes make the skin feel slightly cooler.

Qualifications and training for healing

Anyone can be a healer. Indeed, we all have healing powers. But clearly, when healing is practised professionally there are all sorts of opportunities for crooks and charlatans to take advantage of the innocent. These opportunities are strengthened by the fact that there is no need for special qualifications or training before individuals set themselves up as healers.

Dangers

Apart from the real risk of a patient being taken advantage of by an unscrupulous healer there are no special hazards associated with healing.

The uses of healing

Healing can be used in just about any physical or mental condition. The help of a professional healer is particularly useful in the treatment of conditions where the patient is weary and exhausted and has insufficient energy to use his own self-healing powers without outside support.

Sudden 'miracles' are, naturally, extremely rare. Healing is usually a gradual process. But it is certainly true that a remarkable number of patients do make a recovery after intervention by a healer.

It is perhaps worth mentioning that all the healers I have spoken to insist that healing should be used together with other forms of treatment. Most healers prefer to work alongside orthodox medical practitioners. And, returning the compliment, most orthodox medical practitioners seem happy to work alongside healers.

HEALTH FOODS

The background

A few years ago the phrase 'health food' conjured up images of bean bags, brown rice, kaftans and open-toed sandals. Today the health-food boom has reached a peak. In most developed countries something like 20 per cent of the population is said to patronize health-food shops. In America there is one health-food shop for every 36,000 customers. In Britain the sale of health-food products is worth well over £100 million a year. In Switzerland there is now one health-food shop for every 16,000 inhabitants.

To 'sell' the idea of health food to the public there are now hundreds of health-food experts, wholefood specialists, natural food consultants and journalists anxious to spread the word. There are also dozens of important-sounding committees and organizations dedicated to the promotion of health foods.

These expert committees and advisors claim that health food is more wholesome, that it is free of additives and contaminants, that it has more nutritional value than ordinary food and that specific types of health food can be used to prevent or treat a wide range of dangerous disorders.

Among the specific food products they advocate are substances such as yoghurt, molasses, honey, seaweed, garlic, royal jelly, cider vinegar and ginseng.

The truth I'm afraid is rather different.

For although it is perfectly true that many of the foods sold in supermarkets are either so bereft of nutritional value that they are virtually worthless as foods – or so stuffed with additives, preservatives and pesticide residues as to make them potentially dangerous – the massive and profitable health-food industry has itself created and perpetuated a number of myths.

To begin with the phraseology is often misleading.

So, for example, no one really seems to know what is meant by the phrase 'health food'. All the independent (i.e. not yet 'bought up' by the health-food industry) nutritionists that I've spoken to are just as confused by it as I am. It is, I fear, a quite meaningless phrase which tells you absolutely nothing about the product concerned. The word 'natural' isn't much better either. Butter is a natural food and heroin is a natural plant product. Both have been shown to cause all sorts of damage.

Then there is the phrase 'organically grown' – a phrase which seems to suggest that the food concerned has been reared in some unusually primitive and therefore particularly healthy environment. Once again the fact is that this phrase means absolutely nothing.

The nature of the fertilizer used really has no useful effect on the nutritional quality of a food and many of the products labelled as 'organically grown' contain just as many pesticides and antibiotic residues as anything you're likely to find on the shelves of your local supermarket.

The phrase 'whole food' is rather more useful for it suggests that the food is being sold in its original state – without having had essential nutrients removed from it. But not even this phrase is a guarantee that you can rely on.

The real major problem is, of course, that selling 'health foods' is now very big business. And some people selling 'health foods' are now willing to distort the truth in order to maximize their profits.

To make a diagnosis

Specific health foods are now often sold as treatments for specific disorders. But those who sell health foods for such purposes do not complicate their world by helping their customers to make accurate diagnoses.

The provision of treatment

Many specific health foods are sold as treatments for particular disorders. Ginseng is said to be good for sexual problems. Honey is said to be an excellent tonic. Brewer's yeast is sometimes recommended as a treatment for menstrual or menopausal problems. The links between specific foods and specific conditions do not seem to follow any particular pattern.

Research

Although many companies and individuals now recommend particular foodstuffs for the treatment of named disorders these companies and individuals do not seem anxious to burden themselves with research work.

Many of the alleged treatments are based on what can only be described as 'intuition'.

Qualifications and training for health foods

Health foods are usually sold by individuals who have no training whatsoever. Health foods are often recommended by journalists who have no more training than the shop assistants who sell them.

Dangers

Many of the products sold in health-food stores or recommended by health-food specialists are not particularly safe. Nor are health-food products always good for people. Health-food shops, for example, commonly sell honey as a life-saving food. In fact, honey is simply sugar and is a major cause of tooth decay as well as obesity. The substance called 'sodium chloride' is salt and can cause problems if given to patients who have high blood pressure.

And there are specific dangers too. For instance, there is evidence that patients who have taken laetrile have suffered from cyanide poisoning.

The uses of health foods

There is absolutely no doubt that many of us eat an unhealthy mixture of food. We eat too much animal fat (often as butter, milk and cream rather than as meat), we eat too little roughage and we eat too little fresh food. Too much of the food we eat is over-refined and contains far too many unnecessary additives.

But the sort of products sold in health-food shops are not the answer. For a healthier life we need to eat more fresh fruit and vegetables, eat wholemeal bread and biscuits, less sugar, less butter, less fatty meat, less full-cream milk, less cream and fewer eggs (no more than two or three a week).

HERBALISM

The background

Herbalists can, with considerable justification, claim that theirs is one of the oldest branches of medicine. Animals have instinctively used plants for thousands of years and so have human beings. The use of herbs can be traced back to three thousand years ago in China but I doubt if there has ever been a time when men did not seek comfort from vegetable products of one sort or another. Historians from all around the world have produced evidence to show that all apparently primitive peoples used herbs – often in a sophisticated way.

Penicillin has been used as an antibiotic for thousands of years, rauwolfia has for centuries been recognized as having tranquillizing effects, curare is known as an anaesthetic (it was first used as poison on darts and arrows intended to kill animals and enemies), digitalis is derived from the foxglove and morphine from the opium poppy – both have been widely used for many generations and are still two of the most important drug sources that we know of. Quinine was used to treat the symptoms of malaria long before the disease was identified and the raw ingredients of a common or garden aspirin tablet have been a popular painkiller for far longer than we have had access to tablet-making machinery.

Plants have for centuries been used as aphrodisiacs and contraceptives and there are about three hundred plants which have a fertility-regulating effect – including yam tubers which contain hormone components that form the basis of the modern contraceptive pill.

By the middle of the nineteenth century at least 80 per cent of all medicines were derived from plants, and herbalism *was* practical pharmacology. And then came the revolution inspired by the development of the pharmaceutical industry. Today, in the middle of the 'chemical' era of drugs, only about a third of the drugs we use are plant-based. But herbalism is fighting back – and having a successful revival.

There are several specific reasons for this revival in the fortunes of herbalism – a revival which has been so dramatic that sales of herbal products in the United States of America are now worth a staggering 15 billion dollars a year.

First, there is a massive 'back-to-nature' movement in the Western world – inspired at least in part by the fact that a growing number of people are aware of and frightened of the side effects associated with chemical drugs.

Second, there are many medical disorders (such as arthritis and asthma) that orthodox doctors still cannot cure.

Third, there is a widespread feeling abroad that the individual should retain responsibility for his own health. It is easier to retain responsibility if you are not taking pills which have been prescribed for you by someone else.

Fourth, those who promote and sell herbal remedies have managed to convince their potential customers that herbal remedies are entirely safe. I will deal with this specific claim on page 101.

Whatever the reasons may be for the rise in popularity of herbalism the fact is that there are today millions of people who use herbal products regularly. There are herbal remedies available for just about every illness imaginable – arthritis, menstrual cramps, asthma, bronchitis, coughs, diarrhoea, high blood pressure, anaemia, eczema and dermatitis are just some of the common problems for which herbal remedies are now available.

The herbal remedies are prepared in a variety of different ways. They are available as teas, tinctures, ointments, baths, juices, powders and poultices.

To make a diagnosis

Herbalism is a treatment form. When individuals buy their own herbal remedies they must make their own diagnoses. When herbalists prescribe they rely on guesswork, intuition, iridology, and radionics to help them arrive at a diagnosis.

The provision of treatment

Herbal remedies are taken in two main ways.

First, they can be bought over the counter for use at home – in just the same way as other 'proprietary' medicines can be bought.

Second, they are 'prescribed', and usually 'dispensed', by herbalists.

The main problem with herbal treatments is that there is little continuity and apparently no logic to the type of treatments offered. There are 350,000 known species of plants and about 10,000 of these have been investigated for their medicinal properties. There are some treatment guidelines available to herbalists but most practitioners seem to be rather individual in their choice of remedies.

It is this lack of consistency that really makes herbalism look bizarre and unscientific. In one large book on herbalism, for example, I found a list of twenty-one different substances recommended for patients suffering from eczema. In another major herbal textbook there were eighteen herbal remedies listed for the same condition. Only two of the plants on the second list appeared on the first list. Recommended herbal remedies for eczema have included: great burdock tea, pansy compresses, carrot juice, watercress, comfrey poultices, spinach juice, bergamot oil and strawberry leaf tea.

The practice of herbalism seems even more bizarre when you realize that in many instances herbalists will make up preparations which may contain a mixture of a dozen or more different ingredients. If herbal products do work, and do have potentially powerful effects, then mixing them in this way is at best counter-productive and at worst positively dangerous.

Research

Very few clinical trials have been organized to assess modern herbal products. One of the few properly organized trials concerned a herb called *tripterygium wilfordii*, which grows in the southern part of China and which has for centuries been recommended as a treatment for joint pain. The Institute of Dermatology at the Chinese Academy of Medical Sciences extracted the active principle and found that it worked with moderate success. Unfortunately, like so many other products used for joint pains, the herb was found to produce a wide range of side effects including: gastro-intestinal disorders, blood problems, skin rashes, period problems and sterility.

Qualifications and training for herbalism

There are numerous colleges and institutions which offer training and qualifications for individuals who wish to practise as herbalists. But, sadly, there are many practising herbalists who have far too little knowledge of how the human body works or how herbal products are likely to affect the human body.

Dangers

One of the constant claims made by herbalists is that their products are entirely safe. This is not true. There is now a considerable amount of evidence to show that herbal products can be dangerous.

Recently, for example, the independent Adverse Drug Reaction Bulletin (which is published in England) claimed that herbal medicines can be as toxic as any other drugs and that their reputation for being entirely safe was built in the days when pharmacologists were unaware of the sort of problems that drugs can produce.

It is impossible here to list all the possible side effects of all the available herbal products. But to illustrate the point I am making I have picked out one or two of the commonest herbs and listed some of the side effects known to be associated with their use.

Comfrey Used in the treatment of ulcers, wounds, fractures and hernias. But may cause liver damage and could be carcinogenic.

Evening Primrose Recommended for premenstrual tension, high blood pressure, multiple sclerosis and eczema. But can cause skin rashes, nausea and headaches and should not be given to epileptics.

Feverfew Used in the treatment of arthritis and migraine. But commonly causes mouth ulceration, soreness of the tongue, abdominal pains and indigestion.

Ginseng Commonly used as a sedative and aphrodisiac. Recommended for a huge list of specific problems and as a general tonic. But can cause breast pains, high blood pressure, skin problems, nervousness and diarrhoea.

Hawthorn Used as a sedative and for heart problems and difficulties associated with the menopause. But has a definite effect on the heart and really needs to be taken under medical supervision.

Skullcap Recommended as a diuretic, sedative and tonic. But can cause giddiness, mental confusion and an erratic heart rate.

Valerian Used as a tranquillizer. But can cause giddiness, headaches, spasms, excitability and hallucinations.

Yarrow Used in fevers, colds, high blood pressure and menstrual problems. But can cause headaches, dizziness and skin problems.

All other herbal products also produce their own list of side effects. And when herbs are mixed, as they commonly are, it is nigh on impossible to decide exactly what herb is producing what side effect.

There are two other specific problems that ought to be mentioned here. First, many herbal products react badly with prescribed drugs. Pharmacologists and doctors now firmly recommend that any patient taking a prescribed drug should avoid all herbal preparations. It is, incidentally, also important that patients taking herbal preparations avoid alcohol since some herbs react dangerously with alcohol.

Secondly, there is also a risk that herbal products may be contaminated. So, for example, in 1983 the Department of Health and Social Security in Britain had to issue a warning about a kind of herbal tea made from comfrey leaves. Due to a mistake made somewhere in the packing process the leaves had been contaminated with belladonna (deadly nightshade) leaves. This type of hazard is obviously even greater when local herbalists try preparing their own products or when patients try treating themselves with products they have picked in fields and hedgerows. Even when products are not contaminated it is difficult to judge the purity, quality or strength of an individual batch. Studies of ginseng, for example, have shown tremendous variations in quality and quantity. There are seasonal variations and variations in plants grown in different soils.

It seems clear that in the near future many more dangerous side effects will be recognized as being associated with herbal products. In 1986, for example, the *New England Journal of Medicine* reported that comfrey pepsin capsules, which are widely promoted for the treatment of digestive problems, contain substances which can damage the liver. Anyone taking these capsules for as long as six months runs a real risk of developing serious liver damage.

The uses of herbalism

Despite the enthusiasm of a number of practitioners and uncritical journalists herbalism has no place in twentieth-century medicine. Herbal products are largely ineffective and often dangerous.

HOLISTIC MEDICINE

The background

People often talk about 'holistic medicine' and 'holistic practitioners' as if holism were a speciality like acupuncture or homoeopathy. In fact the word 'holistic' describes an approach, an attitude and a philosophy rather than any specific type of medical practice. A registered medical practitioner working as a family doctor or general practitioner can just as easily practise 'holistic medicine' as can any practitioner of alternative medicine.

The word 'holistic' was first introduced by the South African philosopher and statesman Jan Christian Smuts in *Holism and Evolution* (1926).

Smuts disapproved of the way that scientists and philosophers tried to analyse people and study them as a collection of separate parts. In his book he suggested that the whole human being is much more than (and quite different to) a collection of physical or emotional parts.

The word and the concept lay more or less forgotten until the 1970s when the growth of high-technology medicine led to a revolution among patients and health-care professionals who felt that the modern, aggressive, interventionist approach to healing was quite unsatisfactory.

For over half a century doctors had shown tremendous enthusiasm for specialization. Suddenly there was a widespread feeling that the fragmentation had gone too far. There was also a strong feeling that the 'fragmentation' approach did nothing to help doctors deal with the problems produced by reactions between individuals and their environment.

The consequent search for a more general and more humane approach to health care was nothing particularly new, of course. The Hindus and the Greeks all followed a 'holistic' philosophy several thousand years ago.

But after decades of super-specialization and high-technology medicine the holistic approach seemed new and exciting. The holistic (or wholistic) approach gathered numerous admirers from all sections of society; it brought together psychosomatic medicine (an approach which emphasizes the interdependence of physical and psychological factors), behavioural medicine (in which the psycho-social causes and effects of illness are studied), and humanistic medicine (which emphasizes the importance of a close relationship between the doctor and his patient).

In practical terms this revolution in medical caring meant that instead of regarding patients as sick livers, kidneys or hearts, doctors and other interventionists tried to meet the individual physical, mental, spiritual and emotional needs of their patients. The holistic approach meant that practitioners tried to deal with social and human problems as well as physical ones; that they began to share responsibility with the patient rather than dictating to him; that they tried to use the healing powers of nature and the self-healing powers of the individual and that they tried to spend more time helping patients to understand how psychological processes can be turned into physical symptoms.

The word 'holistic' describes an attitude not a discipline. And it is an attitude that can be shared and enjoyed by orthodox practitioners as well as by alternative practitioners.

To make a diagnosis

The holistic practitioner will use the best diagnostic techniques that are available. If high-technology equipment will improve his or her chances of making an accurate diagnosis – without damaging the patient – then he will use high-technology equipment.

The provision of treatment

Holistic practitioners use many different treatment techniques. They will use drugs when drugs offer the best hope; they will use acupuncture if acupuncture offers the best solution; they will use homoeopathy, surgery or osteopathy. They are truly eclectic in their endeavours. Most important of all they will give precedence to the patient's own natural healing powers.

Research

Since holistic medicine is not a single discipline there are no specific research papers available to show its value. There is, however, a considerable amount of anecdotal evidence available to show that a holistic approach is safe, effective and satisfying both to patients and practitioners.

Qualifications and training for holistic medicine

Any practitioner whose approach is broad-minded, and aimed at dealing with the 'whole' patient rather than parts of him can truly describe himself as an 'holistic practitioner'.

Dangers

There are no specific dangers associated with the practice of holistic medicine. Indeed, on the contrary, the holistic approach is an unusually safe one.

The uses of holistic medicine

In recent years the term 'holistic practitioner' has been abused and misused by thousands of orthodox and alternative practitioners. Orthodox medical practitioners who dabble in acupuncture (after a weekend course) will describe themselves as 'holistic'. Alternative practitioners who use iridology, reflexology and a little herbalism to treat their patients will also describe themselves as 'holistic'.

In reality the genuine holistic practitioner doesn't necessarily have to practise more than one medical discipline. A specialized heart surgeon can be a holistic practitioner just as easily as can a homoeopath. What is important is that the practitioner sees his patient as a whole human being, that he knows the limitations of the type of medicine he himself practises, that he is prepared to refer his patients to practitioners in other disciplines and, most important of all, that he is prepared to allow his patients to share in the responsibility for their own treatment.

HOMOEOPATHY

The background

The principles of homoeopathy go back to the origins of medicine but
the principles of modern homoeopathic practice were established by
Samuel Hahnemann (1755–1843) in the early part of the nineteenth
century.

It was known at that time that cinchona bark (which contains the
drug we now know as quinine) relieves the symptoms of the ague (a
disorder we now know as malaria). In experimental mood
Hahnemann decided to see what happened when he took some
quinine himself – even though he didn't have the ague. He was
startled to discover that when he took the drug he developed the
fever and the other symptoms normally associated with the disease.
In due course he noticed that the symptoms of the disease disappeared when he stopped taking the drug.

Hahnemann knew that according to Hippocrates if an individual
who is suffering from an illness can be made to suffer symptoms
similar to those produced by his illness then he will be cured. This is
the ancient theory of 'like curing like', also known as the law of
similars. Hahnemann realized that quinine satisfied this law and
immediately set about trying to find more drugs that had a similar
effect.

During the following few years he experimented with all sorts of
things: metals, salts, animal products and vegetable substances. He
discovered an enormous range of products which fitted his theory
and which could be used to produce symptoms similar to those
associated with specific disorders.

As he continued his research Hahnemann also discovered

something else: he didn't need to use large doses of his medicines in order to obtain the desired effects. Indeed, on the contrary, to his great surprise he discovered that the smaller the dose he used the more effective it was. And thus the practice of homoeopathy was born.

Minute doses of drugs are given with the intention of triggering off some sort of defensive reaction within the body and stimulating the body's natural resistance to disease. Homoeopathy has, it seems, a good deal in common with vaccination, in which a small amount of an infective organism is introduced into the patient's body in order to stimulate the body's defence mechanisms to prepare suitable defences.

The dilutions that homoeopathic practitioners use are so small that in order to prepare their medicines homoeopathic practitioners effectively empty a bottle of concentrated medicine into a lake and then use the lake water as medicine.

To make a diagnosis

For a homoeopath, making the correct diagnosis is a vitally important part of the whole business of healing. The first interview a patient has with a homoeopath can take as long as two hours. The questions the homoeopath will ask cover a wide range of mental, physical and emotional characteristics, for the homoeopath must find out as much as he possibly can about his patient as an individual. It is only by this lengthy period of questioning that the practitioner can decide what sort of treatment to use because in homoeopathy the treatment is designed to fit the patient not the disease.

The medicine that is to be selected must be one that will suit the patient's psychological make-up, temperament and lifestyle. The homoeopath will be keen to find out what changes the patient has experienced in recent days and weeks. He will want to know about personal feelings and behavioural changes. He will have to know about the patient's needs and fears if he is to choose the correct treatment. The homoeopath will want to know how his patient responds to the temperature, the weather, the environment, and the time of the day.

The homoeopath believes that symptoms are a sign that the body is fighting a danger of some kind. In order to provide the correct treatment the homoeopath needs to know as much as possible about the individual's strengths and weaknesses so that he can provide the correct type of help.

The provision of treatment

In order to evaluate possible treatments homoeopaths have to do 'provings' of potentially useful substances. To do this they must give very small doses of animal, vegetable and mineral substances to healthy people for several weeks. During that time they record any symptoms which are produced.

By his death in 1843 Hahnemann had done 'provings' on 99 substances. By the year 1900 over 600 more medicines had been added to the list of useful remedies. Today there are nearly 3,000 substances which are available to homoeopaths. The materials used include onions, indian hemp, St John's wort, gold, copper, mercury, sulphur, cadmium, honey-bee sting venom, snake venom and spiders.

Once the homoeopath has made his diagnosis then he must choose the correct substance from this list of possible remedies. By and large homoeopaths prefer to use a single cure – however many symptoms the patient has. If, for example, you go to see a homoeopath complaining of a headache and diarrhoea, the homoeopath will probably give you one remedy to treat both problems rather than two separate remedies. The homoeopath always has to remember that it is the patient he is treating – not the disease.

According to homoeopaths there are no incurable diseases, only incurable people.

Over two thousand years ago Hippocrates wrote that 'through the like, disease is produced, and through the application of the like it is cured'. Paracelsus, who was a vital figure in the re-emergence of medicine as a science during the Renaissance, said much the same thing. Hahnemann's basic principle is that 'a substance which produces symptoms in a healthy person cures those symptoms in a sick person.'

Research

There are many mysteries about homoeopathy. How does it really work? How are such diluted medicines able to have any useful effect on the human body? How is it that the more diluted a homoeopathic medicine is the more powerful it seems to be?

There are no answers to these questions. And there do not look like being any answers in the near future. But there is evidence available now to prove that homoeopathy really does work. In the latter part of 1986 British physicians published the results of a double-blind placebo-controlled trial which showed that a homoeopathic remedy significantly reduced the symptoms of hay fever. Other experiments have also provided proof that homoeopathy can work.

It may well be that although future research will confirm that homoeopathy works, researchers will still not be able to provide any acceptable explanation of how it works.

Dr Ronald Davey, a research director of the Blackie Foundation Trust, which was established to try and find out whether or not homoeopathy could be proved to work, has said, 'I am perfectly prepared to accept that ultimately we may only succeed in proving that it is a placebo effect' (i.e. the body heals itself and the practitioner and his treatment act as a catalyst). And Dr Desmond Biddulph, a doctor who practises homoeopathy, has pointed out in a journal written for trainee general practitioners that, 'the physician is the most powerful medicine and the ritual and symbolic interaction between doctor and patient should not be underestimated. The homoeopathic approach exploits this knowledge to the utmost'.

Qualifications and training for homoeopathy

Homoeopathy is practised by fully qualified medical practitioners. It is also practised by many practitioners who have no formal training and no accepted academic qualifications at all. Indeed, homoeopathic remedies are considered so safe that many of them can be bought quite freely without any prescription.

Before visiting a homoeopath it is important to find out whether you are visiting a properly trained medical practitioner – who has spent some years acquiring his skills – or a lay practitioner whose skills may have been acquired from a brief correspondence course.

Dangers

One of the main reasons why Samuel Hahnemann was keen to develop a new form of medical practice was that he was disenchanted by the medicines available to and used by his medical colleagues. (Remember that this was back in the early part of the nineteenth century.) Hahnemann knew only too well that patients were often made worse by being given huge doses of potentially harmful products. He wanted to find a technique that would reduce the risk of patients developing unpleasant or dangerous side effects.

And, indeed, one of the main advantages of homoeopathy over most other forms of medicine (both orthodox and alternative) is that side effects are virtually unheard of.

The only problem that does occur when homoeopathic medicines are used is that the symptoms may sometimes appear to move outwards – producing fresh symptoms such as skin disorders, boils and diarrhoea. These symptoms, claim homoeopaths, show that the treatment is working and that the disease is being eradicated from the body.

The uses of homoeopathy

Homoeopaths are among the most sensitive and cautious of medical practitioners. Most of them, like Hahnemann, have turned to homoeopathy because of a fear of the side effects and dangers associated with modern, powerful drug therapy.

But despite this all good homoeopaths agree that many serious disorders – cancers, serious infections and so on – do need treatment from orthodox practitioners. Homoeopathic remedies should, they claim, be used alongside modern surgical techniques and modern drugs.

Dr Hamish Boyd, Medical Superintendent of the Glasgow Homoeopathic Hospital in Scotland, and one of the world's leading homoeopaths, has stated that 'A good homoeopathic doctor should be a good physician first and then a knowledgeable homoeopath.'

HYDROTHERAPY

The background

Our belief in the healing power of water goes back thousands of years. Many primitive societies believed in the curative powers of Holy Wells and springs and both the Greeks and the Romans believed in the therapeutic value of bathing – indeed, the Roman obsession with public baths was not just due to a yearning for cleanliness or aquatic sports.

After being out of fashion for many hundreds of years, water therapies became fashionable again in the eighteenth century when 'taking the waters' became a popular habit among the wealthy and privileged members of society. All over Europe spa towns flourished (the word 'spa' is taken from the Belgian town of Spa which has been renowned since Roman times for its therapeutic waters). In Germany, France and England spa towns grew ever larger.

Today there are still a number of spa towns throughout Europe that are actively treating patients suffering from a wide range of problems. In France nearly 3,000 treatments a day are given in Vichy alone. In Germany and Italy the jaded, the exhausted and the world-weary still flock to spa resorts such as Baden Baden. In Britain, however, where there are a number of spa towns (at Bath, Buxton, Droitwich, Harrogate, Leamington, Llandrindod Wells, Malvern, Strathpeffer and Woodhall) only the one at Leamington in Warwickshire has continued to function as a proper spa.

The healing power of water is still highly regarded by thousands of practitioners and millions of their patients. The very word used to describe treatment with water – hydrotherapy – does, of course, make the whole thing sound extremely sophisticated. But although hydrotherapy may sound like a science it isn't.

Hydrotherapy can mean drinking water, splashing it onto your body, washing in it, bathing in it, sitting in it, swimming in it and exercising in it. The water can be used cold, warm or uncomfortably hot. It can be delivered by hose, by bucket or by drinking glass. It can be rich with dissolved salts or distilled and pure.

To make a diagnosis

Hydrotherapy is a form of treatment that has no associated diagnostic skills.

The provision of treatment

Hydrotherapy is offered as a form of treatment in many health farms and establishments of a similar type. Patients can sit in cold baths, luxuriate in warm baths where they will be massaged by underwater jets or they can take special showers or underwater massages. The type of treatment offered depends more on the establishment and the patient's personal tastes than anything else.

Research

There has never been any real evidence to show that spa water is particularly good for patients. But there is a considerable amount of evidence to show that some forms of hydrotherapy can help many patients. For example, patients who are immobile because of joint pains, bony injuries or paralysed muscles may be better able to exercise in water where the effects of gravity are minimized.

In addition, the relaxing effects of hydrotherapy can be extremely soothing.

Qualifications and training for hydrotherapy

Patients who visit centres where hydrotherapy is offered for physical problems (such as arthritis or convalescence after a stroke) will usually be guided and assisted by physiotherapists. Physiotherapy is a medical speciality for which special training courses and qualifications are essential.

Dangers

Public baths and jacuzzis can produce or exacerbate urinary problems such as cystitis. Water that is too hot can scald.

The uses of hydrotherapy

If you want a relaxing break then a few days at a spa town or a health farm with a heated swimming pool will almost certainly help you. And if you suffer from joint, bone or muscle troubles then swimming in warm, salty water will undoubtedly prove helpful – although your local swimming pool will probably be much cheaper and just as useful as any of the more expensive establishments.

It is also worth remembering that twenty minutes spent luxuriating in a tub full of warm water can also do both the mind and the body a considerable amount of good. Luxuriating in all-around wet heat will ease aching muscles and soothe the troubled mind. Showers use less water and are more hygienic, and they tend to offer a more stimulating, refreshing bathe.

A final point worth making is that these days a number of manufacturers are selling bottled water as an alternative to tap water. I don't believe that spa-bottled water has any specific properties that are likely to make it especially beneficial to health but those who are worried about the possible contaminants in tap water will be happy to pay for bottled spa water for peace of mind if nothing else.

HYPNOTHERAPY

The background

Hypnotherapy has fascinated men for centuries. It fascinated the Egyptians several thousand years ago and in the seventeenth century a scientific investigator called Athanasius Kircher started to play around with the idea seriously.

But the practice of hypnotherapy really began with Franz Anton Mesmer, an Austrian who graduated in Vienna in 1766. Mesmer believed that human behaviour is controlled by some unseen power from the planets – in much the same way that the moon influences the tides. He argued that this strange power was transmitted via ordinary magnets but after doing a number of experiments he gradually came to the conclusion that the magnets weren't really necessary and that the power could be transmitted – and, more important, controlled – with no physical intermediary at all.

Mesmer soon introduced his idea of 'mesmerism' into popular medical practice and quickly became enormously successful. He was, indeed, so successful that the Austrian medical establishment didn't like him at all and when he went too far by curing a young blind girl they accused him of being a cheat and a charlatan and threw him out of Vienna.

Undeterred Mesmer went to Paris where he established an even more lucrative private practice, using his powerful personality and undoubted presence to attract, dominate and heal his wealthy patients. Unfortunately for Mesmer the French medical establishment didn't like his success either and they decided to get rid of him. In order to make the whole thing look solid and respectable the French set up a commission (which included Benjamin Franklin, one of the signatories of the American Constitution, and Dr Guillotin, who invented the instrument which bears his name) which concluded accurately but unsympathetically that Mesmer's effects were all produced by the imagination.

Mesmer's career was not helped by the fact that the French King Louis XVI had been one of his most enthusiastic supporters. When the French Revolution came Mesmer fled to London.

Since then mesmerism has become known as hypnotism (and known to those who practise it as hypnotherapy) and has suffered a number of setbacks. The first major problem has been that a number of authors have written novels in which hypnosis has been used as an evil force. In *Trilby*, for example, George Du Maurier terrified his readers with the evil character Svengali. Many people still regard Svengali as someone quite real.

The second major problem is that hypnosis has always been popular with stage artistes. This commercialization of the art of hypnosis has undoubtedly had a damaging effect on the status of the associated medical speciality. But slowly, over the years, hypnotherapy has attracted more and more followers. Slowly it has become clear that it can be used to help patients suffering from a wide range of physical and mental problems. Psychiatrists and psychologists have used it and discovered that with its help they can aid patients suffering from a broad variety of anxieties and stress-induced problems.

In addition practitioners have shown that hypnotherapy can be used to delve into the unconscious mind and reveal hidden memories, fears, ambitions and suspicions.

During the last decade or so hypnotherapy has become one of the most popular and fastest growing of all the alternative forms of medicine. It has become big business.

To make a diagnosis

When practised by a skilled expert hypnotherapy can be used to uncover hidden problems and uncover long-forgotten fears. It can be an extremely useful diagnostic technique.

The provision of treatment

Hypnotherapy is normally associated with Svengali-like figures, darkened rooms, drawn velvet curtains, leather couches, soft voices, swinging watch fobs and staring eyes.

Apart from the soft voice none of that is really necessary. Hypnotherapy is, in fact, remarkably easy to practise and anyone who has a reasonably soothing and relaxing voice, and is prepared to spend some time with his patients, can become a skilled hypnotherapist. In order to hypnotize someone you need their trust but very little else.

To be a good subject for hypnotherapy you need to have absolute confidence in the hypnotherapist, you need to be able to relax and you need to want him or her to help you. The more vivid your imagination the more likely you are to benefit. The best subjects for hypnotherapy daydream a good deal and live fairly rich fantasy lives. People who find it difficult to concentrate are difficult to hypnotize whereas individuals who can easily 'lose' themselves in what they are doing are usually fairly easy to hypnotize. It may or may not be of any significance but women are often said to be easier to hypnotize than men.

To induce a hypnotic state the hypnotherapist will usually follow a fairly well-established pattern.

To begin with the patient will need to be sitting or lying comfortably in a room where there are few distractions. A hypnotic state is similar to a sleep state and the sort of physical conditions required for the former are similar to the physical conditions required for the latter.

The hypnotherapist will then begin by talking in a slow, relaxing, confident and controlled manner. He will tell his patient not to worry and he will provide as much reassurance as he possibly can. He may ask his patient to concentrate his eyes on a fixed object such as a pencil or a finger or he may ask his patient to close his eyes and to keep them closed, imagining that his eyelids are getting heavier and heavier.

Next, the hypnotherapist may introduce peaceful images such as green fields, rolling countryside, slow moving streams and so on. Or he may ask the patient to imagine that he is walking down a long staircase.

After fifteen minutes or so of this the patient will be in a light trance – a state half way between waking and sleeping. Gradually over the next few minutes the therapist can usually take the patient into a deeper and deeper trance.

To speed up subsequent consultations the hypnotherapist may plant a suggestion in the patient's mind that will enable him to 'switch on' a trance state much more quickly.

After establishing the trance state the technique used by the hypnotherapist will vary from patient to patient. In some cases the therapist may simply tell the patient that his fears or problems are going to disappear. In other cases he may try to build up the patient's confidence and eradicate long-standing fears.

One of the most sophisticated techniques used by hypnotherapists is regression – a technique in which the therapist takes the patient back through previous months and years in an attempt to unearth problem situations which have led to the development of specific anxieties and fears.

Research

During the last century a considerable number of papers have been published which show the remarkable value of hypnotherapy. Back in 1847 a surgeon called James Esdale performed three hundred major surgical operations in India using hypnosis as the only anaesthetic. Since then evidence has been accumulated to show that by hypnotizing patients, and putting them into an altered state of awareness – somewhere between sleep and wakefulness – it is possible to help combat many different types of pain and discomfort.

Here are details of just a few of the research programmes which have shown the value of hypnotherapy:

1   A paper entitled 'Hypnosis in Terminal Care' which was written by Dr S. O'Connell and published in the *Journal of the Royal Society of Medicine* in 1985 showed that hypnotherapy can be used to help patients who are dying of disorders such as cancer. In such circumstances hypnotherapy helps to relieve pain and other discomfort.
2   A paper entitled 'A Study of Hypnotherapy in General Practice' written by Dr O. Llewellyn Jones and published in *The Practitioner* in 1986 showed that 80 per cent of patients who have been treated with hypnosis are improved in the short term. The long-term success rate was 50 per cent.
3   A paper published in the *American Journal of Clinical Hypnosis* in 1985 showed that hypnotherapy can be used to make warts disappear – even when the warts have been resistant to treatment with liquid nitrogen, curettage and other 'high-technology' techniques.

Those are just three of the research reports which have shown the value of hypnotherapy. There have been many other convincing reports in medical journals all around the world.

It seems, for example, that the body's digestive processes can be controlled by the imagination. In one experiment volunteers were able to produce enzymes which their bodies did not need. Normally, if human beings eat meals that contain a good deal of fat their bodies produce special enzymes which break down the fat and turn it into products which can be readily transported in the blood. Under experimental conditions it was shown that if volunteers were told that they had eaten fat when they hadn't then their bodies would respond to the imagined truth rather than the real truth.

In another experiment it was shown that the body's immune system can be controlled by using the imagination too. Normally when human beings are given an intra dermal tuberculin injection to find out whether or not they are immune to TB their bodies respond automatically. If the individual has been previously exposed to tuberculosis and has prepared internal immune defence systems, a swelling and a small red mark will develop at the site. If the individual has not previously been exposed to TB and has not developed any immune defences no mark and no swelling will develop. This test is done routinely to find out whether patients need vaccinations to help provide them with protection against TB.

And yet researchers have shown that the body's apparently entirely involuntary response to the testing injection can be regulated by the imagination. If an individual who would normally have reacted to an intradermal injection of tuberculin is told not to respond his body does not respond. The swelling and the red mark do not develop. The imagination can, it seems, even control a cell-mediated immunity reaction.

The final, and perhaps most extraordinary piece of research showing that hypnosis can have an effect on the human body was undertaken by Dr Richard D. Willard of the Institute of Behavioural and Mind Sciences in Indiana who asked twenty-two female volunteers, ranging in age from 15 to 54, to use self-hypnosis in an attempt to enlarge their breasts.

At the start of the study, which was eventually described in full in the *American Journal of Clinical Hypnosis*, five individual breast measurements were taken for each woman – circumference, height, width and other measurements were recorded by a doctor who was not involved in the experiments. The volunteers then attended Dr Willard's clinic once a week for six weeks and once every two weeks for an additional six weeks.

At the first session the women were taught how to relax their muscles. Subsequently they were asked to do this and then to imagine that they had a wet, warm towel draped over their breasts. They were asked to imagine that the towel was making their breasts feel warm. If they found this difficult they were asked to imagine that the sun or a heat lamp was shining directly onto their breasts.

At the end of the 12-week experiment 28 per cent of the women had achieved the growth in breast size that they had wanted, 85 per cent had confirmed that a significant increase in their breast size had been achieved and 46 per cent had reported that they had had to buy bigger bras.

When I conducted a similar but loosely structured experiment about three years ago I also obtained impressive results.

Qualifications and training for hypnotherapy

Sadly, as hypnotherapy has become more and more popular – and more and more profitable – thousands of 'specialists' and 'consultants' have set up shop all over the world.

It is possible to take correspondence courses in hypnotherapy – and acquire 'qualifications' – without ever going anywhere near to a patient. I've seen an extended training programme offered which consisted of a two-day seminar. I've lost count of the number of colleges offering training and advising their students on the best way to set up in business.

There are now dozens of institutions, associations, colleges and organizations which claim to represent hypnotherapists. I'm afraid that it is impossible to differentiate between the good, the bad and the terrible.

I recommend that anyone wanting to try hypnotherapy ask their own family doctor for a referral either to a properly qualified psychologist or to a doctor who practises hypnotherapy.

Dangers

There are a number of specific hazards associated with hypnotherapy.

1   The most dangerous technique offered by hypnotherapists who have bought their qualifications cheaply is regression – a technique in which the hypnotherapist claims to be able to take his patient back to his childhood or to a former life.

Scores of hypnotherapists seem to specialize in regression. Some have described their skills in public. But I think this is an exceedingly dangerous 'trick' to try. The main problem is that if a patient under hypnosis is taken back to an unhappy or physically uncomfortable experience then he may become seriously distressed or even physically ill. So, for example, a patient who suffered from bad asthma as a child and who is taken back to his childhood by a thoughtless hypnotherapist may well develop a severe attack of asthma. And that can kill. A patient taken back to

119

a time when he was depressed may well become depressed again.

The other problem with regression is that although scores of the more ignorant therapists in practice argue that they can draw conclusions from the information they obtain, the evidence suggests that what they gather is just a ragbag of miscellaneous, meaningless memories, ideas, feelings, thoughts and snippets of information. Using the information acquired during regression to create useful conclusions is about as sensible as dipping your hand into a dustbin and drawing conclusions about the mental state of the owner from the material you find. It is impossible to differentiate between the useful and the misleading, the relevant and the irrelevant. The hypnotherapist who claims to be able to see patterns in the information he obtains is deluding himself and, worse still, his patient.

2   Hypnotherapists often do not realize that the information they acquire from their patients is not always accurate. Some hypnotherapists seem to believe that anything they are told by hypnotized patients must be the truth. This is not the case. In 1985 the Council on Scientific Affairs of the American Medical Association produced a report in which they showed that recollections obtained during hypnosis can involve confabulations and pseudo memories. They even reported that the material produced during this type of hypnosis is less reliable than information acquired in just about any other way. The reason for this is probably the fact that the brain is far more complex than most hypnotherapists imagine. Many memories are not memories at all but products of the imagination. Hypnosis can too often lead to a type of emotional playtime which reveals dreams and fantasies as well as facts, interpretations, ambitions and regrets as much as genuine memories.

Sadly, many police officers seem to have an unfounded faith in the value of information obtained during hypnosis.

3   Hypnotherapy can easily turn a mild depression into a very serious depression. And yet a number of hypnotherapists who have 'bought' their diplomas claim to be able to treat patients suffering from depression.

4   There is a real risk that patients who are given instructions while under hypnosis may suffer physical damage afterwards. A patient who is frightened of water, for example, may be told, 'You won't be afraid of water in future.' He may then leap into a

lake without first taking the precaution of learning how to swim.

5   There is a danger that by helping a patient to stop smoking or give up overeating a hypnotherapist may take away the patient's much-needed crutch without providing him with an alternative. The patient who smokes to relieve his stress may have a heart attack if he tries to cope with his life without the support of his cigarettes. It is always important to find out why a patient needs a particular crutch before removing that crutch. Remarkably few hypnotherapists seem aware of this simple fact.

6   There is, of course, the risk that a patient may be manipulated by a hypnotherapist. With so many 'quacks' and 'charlatans' practising hypnotherapy this must now be a very real risk.

The uses of hypnotherapy

Good hypnotherapists can help their patients relax, deal with stress and anxiety, get to sleep at night, manage without tranquillizers, drugs or tobacco and deal with panic attacks. Diseases such as asthma, allergy reactions, migraine and eczema respond particularly well to hypnotherapy. Patients who regularly overeat may also be helped by a good hypnotherapist.

ION THERAPY

The background

Most people will admit that just before a storm they feel listless, out of sorts, lethargic and even depressed. After a storm, however, they feel much brighter and fresher.

It is now clear that the explanation for this phenomenon is that before a storm the air around us is heavy with positive ions while immediately after a storm the air contains far more negative ions. It is the positive ions which make us feel low and the negative ions which are stimulating and uplifting.

For some years now researchers have been investigating the influence that the ionization of the atmosphere has on our moods and mental health. Most molecules in the air are neutral but those which carry a charge of some kind are said to be 'ionized'. And it is now generally agreed that negative ions are invigorating while positive ions are debilitating.

To make a diagnosis

Ion therapy is a way of preventing disease – and, sometimes, of treating existing disease. There are no associated diagnostic skills.

The provision of treatment

It is known that a number of factors affect the number of negative and positive ions in the atmosphere – in addition to changes in the weather.

Air-conditioning systems and heating systems, for example, usually increase the number of positive ions in the air while running water (such as is found in a shower) will increase the number of negative ions. This explains why so many people find air conditioning depressing and showers stimulating.

Today it is possible to purchase special small machines which reduce the number of positive ions in the immediate atmosphere and increase the number of negative ions. The main problems with these machines is, of course, that they can only control the ionization of a relatively small volume of air. If doors or windows are opened then the ioniser will not work properly.

Research

A considerable amount of preliminary research has been done to show that increasing the number of negative ions in an atmosphere (and reducing the number of positive ions) has a useful effect on health.

Qualifications and training for ion therapy

There is no need for any special training. The necessary equipment can be bought without a prescription.

Dangers

I know of no specific dangers associated with ion therapy.

The uses of ion therapy

Ionizers, which increase the number of negative ions, are supposed to be good for depression, insomnia, migraine and asthma. They also have a cleansing effect on the atmosphere since negative ions are attracted to pollutant particles (such as cigarette smoke) which they then remove from the air.

It is worth remembering that the number of negative ions in a house can be increased by running a tap or shower while the number of positive ions can be controlled by using central heating and air-conditioning systems sparingly.

IRIDOLOGY

The background

The so-called science of iridology was started in the nineteenth century by a Hungarian doctor called Ignatz Von Peczley who found and nursed an injured owl which had a broken leg. Peczley noticed that the owl had a mark on its eye which disappeared as its leg got better.

On the basis of this single, chance observation, the Hungarian then founded what is now a flourishing branch of alternative medicine. Poets may claim that they can see into your soul by looking into your eyes. Iridologists claim that they can use your eyes to help them check out your body.

Using a torch and a magnifying glass, a special microscope or even a camera with which to take photographs, iridologists will examine their patients' eyes in a search for unusual markings. The iris of each patient's eye is divided into twelve sections – each being related to between five and ten specific parts of your body. According to the markings and colourings that they find iridologists will claim that they can tell what is wrong with patients.

To make a diagnosis

The iridologist examines the patient's eye, maybe even taking photographs of it. With the information he or she has thus obtained he then makes a diagnosis.

The provision of treatment

Iridologists don't offer treatment unless they practise some other therapy. Iridology is purely a diagnostic skill. Occasionally, an iridologist will pass all his patients on to other practitioners – in just the same way as a radiologist will send his patients back to their clinician. More commonly, however, iridologists offer treatment with herbs, acupuncture or some other selected therapy.

Research

I know of no evidence to prove that iridology is of any value whatsoever. The occasional correct diagnosis can easily be explained by the fact that after talking to patients it is often possible to make a good diagnosis. In my view iridology is to medical science what chocolate buttons are to a balanced diet.

Qualifications and training for iridology

Since I consider iridology to be a worthless pseudo science it stands to reason that I consider iridology training to be equally worthless.

Dangers

I know of no specific hazards associated with iridology – unless the practitioner is so clumsy that he pokes out the patient's eye with his magnifying glass or camera.

The uses of iridology

Iridology is one of the few 'alternative' forms of diagnosis. It is, therefore, quite commonly practised by therapists who have no other way of convincing their patients that they know how to make a diagnosis.

In my view iridology is entirely worthless.

KIRLIAN PHOTOGRAPHY

The background

Kirlian photography is named after two Russians called Semyon and Valentina Kirlian who did research on high-voltage photography (or electrophotography) and who suggested that the haloes which their photographs showed around living things provided evidence of the existence of a non-physical energy force or aura.

Those who use Kirlian photography claim that problems or disorders of the body or mind can change the body's powerful electrical force and that these changes can be measured and recorded with their special photographic techniques.

The hands and the feet are, they say, particularly rich in nervous tissue and when high voltage electrical fields are applied to these parts of the body the intensity and size of the interference pattern that is produced will provide the observer with an accurate picture of the physical and mental state of the patient.

Indeed, many practitioners of Kirlian photography go further than this and claim that changes in the patterns of interference occur before there are any physical or psychological signs of illness being present. Kirlian photography is, they claim, an extremely sophisticated and advanced diagnostic aid which enables them to predict future illness patterns.

Kirlian photography is not a new phenomenon. It has been developing for nearly a century. The studies performed by the Russian husband and wife team (the Kirlians) were merely an extension of research which had originally begun at the end of the nineteenth century.

To make a diagnosis

To take his or her pictures the Kirlian photographer places a sheet of photographic paper on a special 'camera' and the patient then puts first a hand and then a foot above the photographic paper. No light source is used but a high-voltage charge is passed across the sensitive paper. The resulting image shows a fringe of light around the object. Once the picture has been developed the Kirlian photographer uses old case histories and specially prepared wall charts to help him 'read' his results.

Kirlian photography is the alternative version of radiology, and photographs taken by Kirlian photographers (sometimes known as practitioners of Kirlian aura diagnosis) are the alternative equivalent of X-rays.

The provision of treatment

Like iridologists Kirlian photographers are diagnosticians. But like iridologists most are prepared to offer some form of treatment or therapeutic advice.

Research

Kirlian photography is in my view primitive and poorly developed. It is neither as efficient nor as widely available as X-ray diagnosis and I know of no solid, scientific evidence to suggest that it has any particular advantages of its own. Professor Ellison of London University, an electronics specialist and a past president of the Society of Psychical Research, claims that the Kirlian effect is simply a product of the body's electromagnetic force.

Qualifications and training for Kirlian photography

Kirlian photography is not widely practised. I suspect that many of those who practise taught themselves – or served an apprenticeship of some sort.

Dangers

I know of no specific hazards associated with Kirlian photography. However, I know of no evidence proving that Kirlian photography is safe.

The uses of Kirlian photography

I do not think it has any.

MACROBIOTIC DIETS

The background

The word 'macrobiotic' is derived from the Greek. 'Macro' means great; 'bio' means vitality and 'biotics' means techniques of rejuvenation.

But although the word is Greek the origin of the diet can be traced back to Japanese Zen monks who chose the diet to satisfy the yin–yang concept of the Tao philosophy.

Those who follow the Tao way of life in order to attain inner peace and good health believe that it is important to obtain a proper balance of yin and yang forces. Yin represents female qualities weakness of character and introversion. Yang represents maleness – extroversion and strength. (These sexist interpretations are not mine – they are derived from original Eastern philosophers.)

The yin and yang philosophy extends into all aspects of an individual's life. Mental activity is a yin force, for example, whereas physical exercise is a yang force. Foods are also classified into yin and yang foods. Yin foods include vegetables, beans, seeds, milk, nuts, fruit and alcohol. Yang foods include eggs, poultry, meat, fish and some powerful tasting foods such as ginger. Rice is considered neither specifically yin nor specifically yang.

The nutritional system of the Zen macrobiotic diet is based on ten ways of eating (and drinking) which are numbered on the scale − 3 to + 7. There are in other words ten separate macrobiotic diets. The five lowest diets allow the consumption of some animal foods but the higher diets allow only a vegetarian diet. At the highest stage only cereal is allowed. Even water consumption must be kept to an absolute minimum.

The aim is that the individual who follows a macrobiotic diet should start with the least restrictive diet and slowly work his way up to the most restrictive diet – until he is existing on a few cereals and little else.

To make a diagnosis

The macrobiotic diet is a way of life and there are no diagnostic skills associated with it.

The provision of treatment

The macrobiotic diet is a way of life intended to provide those who follow it with a healthy, happy mind and body.

Research

The macrobiotic diet is based on religious and philosophical principles rather than science.

Qualifications and training for macrobiotics

No qualifications or training are required.

Dangers

The simpler, less restrictive macrobiotic diets are quite healthy and contain a good mix of foods. But the more restrictive macrobiotic diets are extremely dangerous and those who follow them run a real risk of developing a nutritional deficiency.

Problems that have been reported among patients following the more restrictive diets include: scurvy, anaemia, dehydration and emaciation. Special problems can occur when babies and small children are fed on a macrobiotic diet. The amount of available protein is likely to be too low and the baby or child is also likely to develop serious vitamin and mineral deficiencies. Rickets has been reported among children following a macrobiotic diet. The macrobiotic diet has been condemned as a threat to human health and parents who impose the diet on their children have been accused of child abuse.

The uses of a macrobiotic diet

None that I know of – apart from whatever philosophical satisfactions the individual may obtain from following the diet.

MASSAGE

The background

Massage has been popular for thousands of years and is of more value than most of us imagine. In recent years postcard-sized advertisements in seedy shop windows have given massage a rather bad name. However, massage can help ease tension, soothe tight muscles and relieve pain extremely effectively. Massage helps in a number of quite specific ways.

First, it helps to clear away the knots that accumulate in your muscles when you are tense or anxious. Normally when you feel tense your muscles tighten as part of your natural response to stress and fear. Your body responds in this way because it assumes that a physical response will help you deal with your stress – indeed, if you are facing a genuine physical threat then it will help if your muscles are ready for action: you'll be better able to run, jump, climb or fight.

Unfortunately, of course, most of our problems these days can't be dealt with by a purely physical response. And so the physical response is inappropriate. Even more important is the fact that as your problems and worries and tensions persist, so does your muscle tension. And as the tension persists so the muscles stay contracted and waste products such as lactic acid accumulate. These accumulated wastes worsen things by making your muscles stiff and painful and preventing them from relaxing.

By massaging these areas (and most commonly muscle tension seems to affect the muscles in the neck, shoulders and back) it is possible to clear away the accumulated wastes, and to relieve muscle stiffness. A good massage can clear knots out of muscles just as surely as it is possible to clear the wrinkles from a bed sheet by gentle stroking.

Second, the personal contact that is an inevitable part of a massage helps too. In our society we touch one another comparatively little; social rules and requirements make it unacceptable for us to touch strangers or even to touch loved ones in public. And yet there is a good deal of evidence to show that we need to be touched and to touch one another. Children who are not cuddled or touched by their parents as they are growing up will develop all sorts of emotional problems – the same thing happens with young animals too. Gentle massage can help relieve pain and tension by providing sympathy and reassurance.

Third, there are some doctors and psychologists who believe that by relaxing muscles through massage a masseur doesn't just have an effect on the body but has a very positive soothing effect on the mind too. Wilhelm Reich, a psychologist who practised earlier in the century (see page 60), believed that some people hide their emotions in their muscles and that there is a strong link between the two. Just what the link consists of is a mystery but it is certainly true that many people do feel mentally relaxed and comfortable after a massage.

Finally, and perhaps most important of all, there is evidence that massage has two very specific and positive pain-relieving effects. It helps to stimulate the production of endorphins, the body's internally produced pain-relieving hormones. And by stimulating the production of sensory impulses which will be carried along the body's larger nerve fibres it blocks the transmission of pain messages by closing the gate at the spinal cord.

An additional advantage is that when you are able to move your muscles and joints more freely after massage your brain will start sending instructions down your spinal cord to your muscles; those descending impulses also play a part in keeping the spinal cord gateway closed to pain impulses.

To make a diagnosis

It is important to know what is wrong before having a massage. Otherwise there is a danger that a minor problem may be turned into a major problem. However, most masseurs and masseuses have few diagnostic skills. By and large it is up to the patient to decide whether or not his problem requires more skilled medical attention.

The provision of treatment

It is possible to obtain a good massage in most towns or cities these days. Most health farms or large hotels can give you the name and telephone number of a reliable local masseur. Health clubs, swimming baths and gyms are another possibility. Or you could pick a name out of the Yellow Pages of the telephone directory or the advertisements in your local newspaper. But do make it clear why you want a massage, and remember that a 'relief massage' is something quite different.

It is important, too, to remember that there is a tremendous difference between massage and manipulation. The former simply involves the rubbing, kneading and rolling of the skin and muscles. The latter involves stretching and twisting joints.

And you should also remember that massage should never be painful, although when relieving stiffness it may occasionally prove slightly uncomfortable. If you're having a massage and it hurts, then tell the masseur to stop and be more gentle.

Finally, it is worth remembering that although a professional massage can be extremely pleasant you don't have to visit a professional in order to benefit from a massage: you can simply persuade a friend or relative to give you one.

For a home massage you should follow these simple instructions:

1   Make sure that you both feel completely comfortable. Any clothes that either of you wear should be loose and light and the room temperature should be pleasantly warm. If the temperature is too low your muscles will contract and become stiff and difficult to massage. The room should not be too light, so simply use a small bedside lamp or table lamp for illumination. You may both find gentle background music helpful and relaxing.

2   Although a massage couch is obviously ideal, very few homes have anything comparable to the equipment likely to be available in a professional's clinic or studio. A bed or springy sofa will be useless, since there will be far too much bounce in either. The most satisfactory solution is for the person who is to have the massage to lie down flat on the floor. A foam mat or a couple of rugs spread out on the carpet should be enough to make things acceptably comfortable. If you're going to use oil or powder during the massage then it is a good idea to spread an old sheet over the carpet to catch the mess.

3   If you're going to have your back massaged you won't need any cushions but if you're going to have the front of your body massaged put one small cushion under your head and another under your knees.

4   Remember that oil lubricates the skin and makes it much easier

132

to give a massage. (If you don't like oil then use talcum powder which works almost as well.) You can buy very light, easily absorbed massage oils. (You can use scented oils if you fancy the idea – see aromatherapy on page 42 – but I don't believe it will make any difference to the effectiveness of the massage.)

5 The individual giving the massage should just follow his or her intuition. Start with a general massage involving all areas of the body and concentrate your massage attempts on those specific parts of the body which are particularly sore or tense. Be cautious when moving joints and avoid the spine completely. When giving a massage it often helps to be quite firm with the kneading and pummelling.

Research

I know of nothing other than anecdotal evidence to support the value of massage.

Qualifications and training for massage

There are courses for those who would masseurs be. But as long as your masseur is careful, clean and courteous I don't think you need worry too much about qualifications.

Dangers

As long as the masseur does nothing that is painful and avoids joints and the spine and infected areas then he is unlikely to do any harm.

The uses of massage

Massage is very good for sore and painful muscles. It is also extremely relaxing and an excellent way to deal with the problems produced by stress and anxiety.

MEDITATION

The background

Under normal everyday circumstances an almost unending stream of facts and feelings pour into your mind. Your eyes and your ears join with your other senses in gathering an enormous variety of bits and pieces of information. Each one of those pieces itself produces assessments, interpretations and conclusions. Even when you aren't consciously thinking of anything, or putting yourself under pressure, thousands of sensory messages keep your body busy adapting to changes in your environment.

During the last few decades scientists in a number of very reputable institutes around the world have produced evidence to show that if you can cut down the amount of information that your mind is receiving then you will cut down the number of mental responses that take place. You will become rested and relaxed and your body and your mind will benefit in a number of positive ways. If you suffer from any stress-induced disorders (such as high blood pressure, colitis, asthma, indigestion or eczema for example) you will benefit enormously. If you suffer from any stress-induced mental problems (such as anxiety or insomnia) that problem will also diminish in importance. And you will benefit by feeling stronger and healthier and by being more resistant to disease and disorders of every kind.

Unhappily, of course, many people find it very difficult to relax properly. We feel guilty if we slow down. We feel that we are failing ourselves and those around us if we sit and watch the world go by for a minute or two. We've been conditioned to think that only by pushing ourselves as hard as possible will we ever achieve anything worth while or win the respect of those around us. We are used to our lives being fast and frenetic and we regularly push ourselves too far and too quickly. We do not allow ourselves time to unwind; and we do not allow ourselves the chance to soothe our minds (and therefore our bodies) with pleasant, gentle, relaxing images.

We try to relax, of course. But many people assume that if they sit down in front of the television set with a sandwich and a beer they are relaxing. In fact, of course, that sort of relaxation may help the body but it doesn't help the mind very much. Lying down in a stupor in front of the television won't do very much to soothe a troubled mind. The images and memories of the day's problems will continue to fight for space alongside the images being projected by the evening's television programmes. The television news will be full of terrible new worries to be added to the ones already clamouring for attention.

Meditation became popular when it became clear that although relaxation is important it is something that a lot of people find difficult to do. Derived from centuries-old Eastern practices, meditation was first investigated in the early 1970s. In 1972, for example, two American researchers, Robert Keith Wallace and Herbert Benson, published results which showed that during meditation an individual's metabolic rate and oxygen consumption will both fall. Wallace and Benson (one of whom was an Assistant Professor of Medicine at Harvard Medical School) showed that people who meditate become calmer and less anxious than people who don't.

All around the world other physiologists and doctors came up with similarly impressive results. In Britain it was shown that during meditation the blood pressure falls noticeably. In France it was shown that people who meditate can learn to slow their heart rate. In Germany it was shown that people who learned to meditate could deal more effectively with anxiety and depression. It was shown that individuals who learned these skills could control their body temperatures and breathing rates.

Of course, there was nothing really new in any of this. The repetitive dance and chant rhythms used by primitive tribes all around the world have always been used to produce a loss of self-awareness and an accompanying sense of soothing relaxation. For years it has been known that Eastern mystics can stop their hearts at will.

But suddenly meditation became very popular. Many people saw it as the answer to stress. Experts like the Maharishi Mahesh Yogi (the man who was known as the guru followed by the Beatles and whose type of meditation is known as 'transcendental meditation') were everywhere – on television talk shows, in newspapers, in magazines. Meditation as practised for centuries by followers of Eastern religions became very big business.

It really didn't work. Even though many doctors quickly accepted that meditation helps by triggering off the body's own quite natural relaxation response – the natural antithesis to the stress response – the majority of those who might have benefited from meditation never really took to it. And stress problems continued to kill thousands every year.

There are, I think, several reasons why formally organized meditation never caught on in the West.

First, and most important, the religious and semi-religious features which were seen as an essential part of many forms of meditation were seen as frightening and forbidding by many people. The words 'relaxation' and 'meditation' became linked with shaven-headed mystics, religious groups and orange-robed eccentrics. People wanted to know how to deal with life. Instead they were offered a bizarre escape route. They didn't want to take part in organized rituals and they knew that they would feel self-conscious if they had to sing or chant any magic incantations.

Mantras, contemplative techniques and imagined paradoxes ('imagine that you can hear one hand clapping') are just some of the consciousness expanding techniques favoured by those who teach traditional meditation techniques.

Many who tried to introduce meditation into the Western culture made the simple mistake of trying to introduce a technique devised for an Eastern culture – a technique quite unsuitable for mass marketing in the Western world.

Even when meditation was adapted for Western minds it was too often turned into something fearfully pretentious. So, for example, consider this quote from a brochure advocating a form of meditation known as 'conscious breathing':

'Through a simple process of connecting your inhale to your exhale in a loving safe environment you connect to your own highest source of life.'

What nonsense!

It's hardly surprising that millions backed away from meditation and relaxation and refused to have anything to do with these theories.

The second major problem was that many of those who talked of the value of meditation claimed that in order to benefit, people had to empty their minds of all inputs and all thoughts. That really isn't easy. And many people found the prospect of completely emptying their minds so daunting that they didn't even try.

As a result meditation has remained relatively unpopular, the perogative of a small number of individuals.

To make a diagnosis

Meditation is a form of treatment. There are no associated diagnostic skills.

The provision of treatment

Formal programmes of meditation follow fairly strictly structured plans. The patient will be told to sit in a special position, empty his mind, repeat a particular phrase over and over again and maintain the position and the chant for many minutes, even hours, at a time.

There is no doubt that such formal programmes do work. But as I have already pointed out, millions of Westerners find meditation difficult to accept or practise. And for them there are simpler 'westernized' alternatives which are far more acceptable and yet just as effective. For example, in my books *Bodypower* and *Mindpower* I recommended the techniques which I call 'daydreaming'.

Most of us daydream when we are small. But our teachers and our parents teach us that it is a wasteful, undesirable habit that we must lose. In fact it isn't a bad habit at all. It is, on the contrary, a natural technique which can help you relax your mind thoroughly and achieve a beneficial level of tranquillity even when things around you are just as hectic as ever. When you daydream you use a cut-out process which your mind has available but which it has forgotten how to use.

To daydream effectively you have to allow your imagination to dominate your thinking and to take over your body too. It really isn't a difficult trick to master and once you've learned how to do it you'll be able to use the technique wherever you happen to be and whatever you happen to be doing. (Although I must warn you that the daydreaming technique is so effective that you should not try it while driving or operating machinery of any kind.)

To begin with you have to learn how to practise. Learning to daydream is a bit like learning to play golf or learning how to dance. If you don't practise it will never come easily or naturally.

Start by finding somewhere comfortable to lie down. Your bedroom is probably the best place. Close the door and lock it if you can. Put a 'Do not disturb' notice on the outside door handle. Before you go into your room, by the way, take the telephone off the hook, put the cats out and make sure that there isn't anyone due to call or arrive home for fifteen or twenty minutes or so.

Now, lie down on your bed and make yourself as comfortable as you can get. Take big, deep breaths and try to conjure up some particularly restful and relaxing scene from your past. Don't let anyone wander into your daydream because if you do then the chances are that your daydream will either become a fantasy or a nightmare.

You can, of course, use just about any scene you like when you are daydreaming. And you can even build up a library of your own private, favourite daydreams.

Some of your daydreams can be based on real memories. Some can be memories taken from films, television programmes or radio programmes. Some may be based on scenes you've encountered in favourite books or magazines.

If you find it difficult to create your own daydream images then hunt out an old photograph or postcard of a spot that you remember as being restful, peaceful and relaxing. Carry the photograph with you and look at it through half-closed eyes as often as you can. Try to imagine yourself there once again. Try to remember all the relevant sensations: the sounds, the smells, the temperature and so on. Try to see yourself in that relaxing situation as often as you possibly can.

In future when you go on holiday collect postcards of the places that you find comfortable and calming. Take your own photographs too and if possible get someone to take photographs showing you sitting or lying somewhere peaceful, comfortable and relaxing. Then carry the postcards and photographs around with you.

Daydreaming has one important advantage over the type of meditation favoured by religious groups. With meditation you have to empty your mind completely and replace real anxieties and troubles with a clinically empty, clean space. That isn't easy to do. When you daydream you replace your natural fears with calming, comfortable, tranquil memories which do themselves have a useful and positive effect.

Meditation does, undoubtedly, halt the damage caused by the pressures of the outside world. But when you fill the void instead with peaceful, tranquil thoughts, you don't just halt the damage – you do much more. You can build up your inner strength by filling your mind with positive health-giving feelings. Once you have learned how to daydream properly then you will be able to use the same technique just about wherever you are and whatever you are doing. If you're stuck in a traffic jam, for example, and you feel your heart rate rising and your muscles tensing, just lie back and get as comfortable as you can. Close your eyes and imagine that you are on your beach or in your country hotel. Replace the real fears and frustrations of the world around you with the relaxing feelings and memories of a scene that you find soothing and calming.

Similarly you can try the same technique when you are sitting in an office and beseiged by people anxious for your attention. Take a few minutes off and rest completely and properly. If there is nowhere else to do your daydreaming disappear into the washroom. A few minutes' relaxation will help you work far more effectively and efficiently.

Incidentally, if you want to prove to yourself just how useful this technique can be, take your pulse when you start a daydreaming session and then take your pulse again when you finish. You'll almost certainly find that your pulse rate will fall noticeably during a ten- or fifteen-minute daydreaming session.

Research

There is a considerable amount of published research available in the world's medical and scientific journals which shows the value of meditation in any one of its many forms. At the last count there were over 350 different scientific papers proving that this type of therapy really does work.

Meditation has been shown to reduce high blood pressure, reduce the need for treatment for conditions such as anxiety and depression, help heal asthma, headaches, allergies and skin problems, help patients with diabetes, help patients diet successfully, help patients manage without cigarettes or alcohol, help reduce accidents, help people get to sleep and help patients maintain good physical and mental health.

Meditation – in whatever form it is used – is probably the most important, and most underestimated, healing technique available to us.

Qualifications and training for meditation

If you want to learn transcendental meditation then you will need to attend special classes where you will be taught by lecturers who have knowledge of the subject. Other types of meditation are often taught at colleges and schools all around the world. The daydreaming technique which I have described needs no special training and no special qualifications.

Dangers

After relaxing through either formal meditation or daydreaming you should not get up too quickly. If you have relaxed efficiently your blood pressure will have fallen fairly considerably. And if you do get up too quickly you'll probably feel rather dizzy. Instead, stretch your arms and legs carefully and gently for a minute or two. If you've been lying down move slowly into a sitting position and stay like that for a few seconds in order to give your body time to adapt.

The uses of meditation

Meditation (or daydreaming) will help you improve your resistance to pressure and reduce your susceptibility to the many disorders now known to be caused by too much stress.

MUSIC THERAPY

The background

The Indians were probably the first to recognize the value of music therapy. Four thousand years ago Hindu doctors used to play soothing gentle music while surgeons were operating. They used to play music in the wards too. They discovered that music helped people to relax and get better quicker.

Only in the last few decades, however, have we relearned the truth about the healing power of music. Thirty years ago in Scotland a psychiatrist called Dr Isaac Sclare used music, and in particular violin playing, to help patients suffering from a wide range of mental disorders. And since then the value of music therapy has been proven on many occasions. An Italian doctor has demonstrated the value of various forms of music in the treatment of mental and emotional problems and for several years now it has been possible for students at the Catholic University of America in Washington DC to study for a master's degree in music therapy.

From the evidence now available it seems clear that music can be soothing and relaxing. It can cheer people up when they are sad. It can calm them down when they are anxious or over-excited. It can help people move about when they are stiff or uncomfortable. It can bring back happy memories to people who are troubled by depression and despair. And it can help relieve pain.

You don't even have to be conscious to benefit from music therapy. Research at the Special Care Baby Unit at Dorset County Hospital in England has shown that playing a tape of pulsating simple sounds almost continuously helps ensure that premature babies stay alive. Music can, it seems, penetrate and benefit the mind that is deaf to conversation.

To make a diagnosis

Music therapy is a form of treatment. There are no associated diagnostic skills.

The provision of treatment

A music therapist will help choose music for you – or teach you how to play an instrument. But you don't really need any outside advice to help you decide which types of music you find most soothing, relaxing, calming or invigorating. Once you have decided on the types of music that you find most therapeutic, keep the appropriate records or tapes around so that you can use them when you need them.

Some people find classical music most relaxing. Others prefer hard rock music. Many seem to find soothing, traditional ballads most calming. A portable cassette recorder with a pair of headphones will enable you to enjoy your favourite music wherever you are, without annoying your neighbours. You are also likely to find it easier to 'lose' yourself in your music if you use headphones.

And don't forget that you can benefit by playing music as well as listening to it. The piano and the guitar seem to be the instruments most likely to prove soothing.

Research

A surprising amount of research has been published to substantiate claims that music therapy is effective. In one of the most remarkable experiments conducted to show the pain-relieving value of music Drs M. Borzecki and K. Zakrzewski of the Pain Clinic at the Warsaw Academy of Medicine used music to help seventeen patients suffering from backache, headaches and trigeminal neuralgia. They found that music had an extremely valuable effect on their patients and helped to control even quite savage pains.

In another experiment, reported in *The Practitioner*, 1984, Dr T. Goroszeniuk and Barbara M. Morgan of Queen Charlotte's Hospital for Women in London showed that a high proportion of women undergoing Caesarian section under epidural anaesthesia benefited from listening to music played through a portable cassette player fitted with headphones.

Qualifications and training for music therapy

Although it is possible to obtain a degree in music therapy this does seem to me to be one speciality where training and qualifications are superfluous.

Dangers

I cannot imagine any hazards that could be associated with music therapy – assuming, of course, that the patient is not subjected to music to which he has a strong aversion.

The uses of music therapy

Music therapy helps patients relax, move more easily, forget their pain and overcome mental problems such as depression. It is a remarkably effective and extremely safe form of therapy which is widely under-used.

NATUROPATHY

The background

Naturopathy was undoubtedly founded by Hippocrates who, around 400BC, said that the best way to maintain good health was to eat and exercise moderately and carefully. According to Hippocrates nature heals extremely effectively and the body can look after itself very well.

In the nineteenth century these simple concepts were adulterated slightly when naturopaths started to use herbal remedies – on an empirical rather than a scientific basis.

Today naturopaths follow three basic guiding principles.

First, they believe that all forms of disease are caused by the accumulation of waste products within the body and that these products accumulate because of bad living habits.

Secondly, they believe that the body is always striving for the ultimate good of the individual and that when symptoms do appear they merely indicate that the body is trying to deal with a problem.

Thirdly, they claim that the body contains within itself the power to deal with illness.

The second and third of these principles are undoubtedly sound. The first is much more controversial and less well-founded on fact.

To make a diagnosis

Naturopaths use a variety of diagnostic techniques. One of the most commonly favoured techniques is iridology (see page 124). Since

144

naturopathy is, by and large, founded on good sense this is rather a pity.

The provision of treatment

Most naturopaths begin their work by trying to persuade their patients to change their bad eating habits. Usually they will start treatment by recommending a complete fast to help the body get rid of all the poisonous substances and unwanted wastes that it contains. Then they will encourage their patients to leave out all junk foods and foods that contain stimulants, foods that are rich in additives and foods that contain large amounts of fat or sugar. It is perhaps worth mentioning that naturopaths have for many years been recommending high-fibre diets and were among the first practitioners to point out the existence of allergy problems caused by pollutants in the food we eat.

In addition to these rules about food and eating, naturopaths will recommend relaxation exercises, physical exercises, osteopathy, massage, hydrotherapy, fresh air, vegetarianism, vitamin supplementation and many other treatment techniques.

Research

The main basic principle of naturopathy is that the human body knows best and that it should be given a chance to heal itself. The guiding principle is that the patient should be taught self-awareness and independence. My book *Bodypower* contains a large number of scientific references which support these twin theses and which substantiate the claim that the body's self-regulating mechanisms are capable of dealing with a wide range of disorders.

Qualifications and training for naturopathy

There are many courses and diplomas available for those who wish to practise naturopathy. Some of these courses are quite exhaustive; others are extremely superficial.

Dangers

There are no specific dangers associated with the practice of naturopathy although, naturally, when specific techniques and treatments are used then there may be hazards.

The uses of naturopathy

The naturopathic approach to healthy living is a common-sense one which highlights the virtues of sensible living and moderation in all things. Inevitably, patients who follow the principles of naturopathy will occasionally need outside help from health specialists. It is a pity that the purity of naturopathy has been contaminated by its association with quack remedies and charlatanism.

OSTEOPATHY

The background

Some osteopaths trace their profession back hundreds of years from the simple, roving surgeons of early times and through the bone setters of the eighteenth century. It was not, however, until the year 1874 that the founder of modern osteopathy, Andrew Taylor Still, announced his theories about health and medicine.

Still was an American, the son of a methodist preacher, and he hated drugs and alcohol of all kinds. He firmly believed that the human body can be treated as a machine and that faults in the musculo-skeletal system are responsible for the development of a huge variety of diseases. Although one of Still's early students, a man called John Martin Littlejohn, tried to expand the basis upon which osteopathy was founded, most of Still's followers believed that they could help their patients best by manipulating their spines.

Today, although a small number of osteopaths will claim that they can help deal with a much wider range of problems, the majority of practising osteopaths concentrate on dealing with backache, leg pains, headaches and neck pains by manipulating bones and joints. Indeed, the figures suggest that well over 50 per cent of all the patients going to an osteopath have one particular type of problem: backache.

To make a diagnosis

Osteopaths diagnose their patients by watching the way that they walk, stand and sit; by taking a full personal history; by performing a physical examination and by taking X-rays.

The provision of treatment

Osteopaths usually treat their patients with massage and manipulation of various kinds. They stretch and move their patients' joints and they perform 'high velocity' thrust techniques.

There is an additional type of osteopathy – cranial osteopathy – that ought to be mentioned here. Pioneered by a nineteenth-century osteopath, William Sutherland, cranial osteopathy is used both to help make a diagnosis and to help in treatment. Sutherland was interested in the structure of the skull and after study he decided that all twenty-two bones of the skull could be moved by manipulation. He believed that by gentle touch and pressure the skull could be realigned and that a slight pressure from the therapist's hands on the patient's head could prove extremely relaxing.

Research

Surprisingly little research has been done to illustrate the value (or lack of value) of osteopathic treatment. Most of the available evidence is anecdotal.

Qualifications and training for osteopathy

There are a remarkable number of colleges and training establishments offering courses and diplomas for would-be osteopaths. In Britain, for example, there are The Society of Osteopaths, the British Osteopathic Association, the Osteopathic Medical Association, the British Naturopathic and Osteopathic Association, the General Council and Register of Osteopaths (which sounds more official than it is), the Andrew Still College of Osteopathy and Natural Therapeutics, the British School of Osteopathy, the European School of Osteopathy, the London College of Osteopathic Medicine, the British and European Osteopathic Association, the Cranial Osteopathic Association, the Natural Therapeutic and Osteopathic Society and Register, the Osteopathic Association of Great Britain and undoubtedly several more.

Most of these are in competition with one another. It is hardly surprising that patients find it extremely difficult to differentiate between the competent and the incompetent.

Dangers

Osteopaths often claim that osteopathy is completely safe. It isn't. The manipulation of joints can lead to problems. So, for example, the journal *Laryngoscope* recently contained a report of a 29-year-old woman who visited an osteopath and suffered sudden sensorineural hearing loss following manipulation of her cervical spine.

Osteopathy is a potentially hazardous procedure that needs to be carried out with great care. It should only be used after a thorough diagnosis has ruled out the possibilities of there being some condition (such as a fracture, a tumour or an infection) which makes manipulation unwise.

The uses of osteopathy

Osteopathy is an excellent form of treatment for simple bone, joint and muscle problems. Most doctors with backache visit osteopaths or chiropractors.

PENDULUM DEVICE

The background

A small, heavy bob on a piece of string is the basis of this so-called diagnostic aid. Made of wood, plastic or metal the bob looks rather like a builder's plumb-line.

The operator (usually called a 'dowser') swings the pendulum and then puts a question to it. Eventually the pendulum will start to move in a circular fashion. In advance the 'dowser' will have decided which direction – clockwise or anticlockwise – means yes and which means no.

To make a diagnosis

The question is asked, the pendulum is swung and a 'yes' or 'no' answer will be provided.

The provision of treatment

I hate to think what treatment techniques pendulum dowsers might recommend.

Research

None.

Qualifications and training for pendulum device control

None.

Dangers

Believing in it.

The uses of the pendulum

It can be used to define the direction of gravity and in general building work.

PSYCHIC SURGERY

The background

Psychic surgery is a technique commonly used in Brazil and in the Philippines for the removal of diseased tissue and tumours from the body of a patient.

To make a diagnosis

Practitioners don't waste time with diagnoses.

The provision of treatment

The practitioner will move his hand over and around the patient's body and will then suddenly produce a piece of diseased and bleeding flesh. This, he will show to the patient as evidence that some internal badness has been removed.

Research

Research has shown that the tissue these practitioners remove is invariably of animal origin.

Qualifications and training for psychic surgery

Practitioners are presumably trained for the ordinary theatre rather than the operating theatre. Membership of the Magic Circle is probably useful.

Dangers

It is possible to develop skin rashes and infections from offal.

The uses of psychic surgery

Entertainment.

PSYCHOPERISTALTIC MASSAGE

The background

Psychoperistaltic massage (which is also known as biodynamic massage) was devised thirty years ago by Gerda Boyesen, a Norwegian-born psychologist and physiotherapist. Boyesen is a follower of Wilhelm Reich (see page 60) and is said to accept his claim that the body knows as much as the mind and that pain is simply trapped energy.

   While working as a physiotherapist Boyesen decided that the trapped energy that causes pain exists as fluid embedded between muscles and nerves. She then discovered that by massaging the body it is possible to liberate the energy-rich fluids.

To make a diagnosis

Psychoperistaltic massage seems to be a form of treatment. I know of no allied diagnostic skills.

The provision of treatment

Treatment is provided by massaging specific parts of the body.

Research

I have not been able to trace any.

Qualifications and training for psychoperistaltic massage

It is possible to be trained in psychoperistaltic massage.

Dangers

I doubt if there are any specific dangers with this type of treatment.

The uses of psychoperistaltic massage

I doubt if there are any.

PSYCHOTHERAPY

The background

The word 'psychotherapy' must be one of the most misunderstood and abused in our language. Strictly speaking it simply means 'treatment of the mind'. But under that broad, apparently respectable definition, there lies an enormous number of doubtful techniques and unreliable practices.

To make a diagnosis

As with many other specialists psychotherapists 'diagnose' their patients by listening to them.

The provision of treatment

To a large extent the treatment is in the listening. Most psychotherapists seem to make up treatment techniques of their own. One psychotherapist's way of encouraging patients to learn self-control is to order them to refrain from sex for a year. Another psychotherapist tells bulimic patients that they have to give him money every time they vomit. The first time they have to pay a penny. They have to double the sum on each subsequent occasion. 'Patients soon work out that it is going to cost them a fortune if they keep going – so they stop,' says the therapist, who charges a fee for this 'treatment'.

Research

No controlled trials have ever been done to assess the value of psychotherapy.

Qualifications and training for psychotherapy

Anyone can set up a 'surgery' or a 'clinic' as a psychotherapist. You do not need any formal qualifications. In America a pet chameleon was licensed as a psychotherapist.

Dangers

It has been shown that most patients who see psychotherapists are overtly manipulated by their therapists. Many patients are abused (sexually or financially or both).

The uses of psychotherapy

All the available evidence suggests that patients are as likely to benefit from talking to a friendly barman or taxi driver as they are from talking to a 'qualified' psychotherapist (or psychoanalyst). A talk to a sympathetic friend or hairdresser will do just as much good as a talk to a psychotherapist. In most cases it will probably do far more good.

RADIONICS

The background

Radionics is a method of diagnosis based on a theory of electro-magnetic energy flow that was devised by Albert Abrams (1863–1924) of San Francisco. Abrams claimed that diseased tissue produces electromagnetic radiation and that the disease process can be reversed by beaming back a corrective flow of radiation.

Those who have used the radionics 'black box' devised by Abrams have put forward several explanations as to how it works. But the credibility of radionics as a medical speciality was damaged when it was found that many practitioners didn't bother to connect their black boxes to any power source.

To make a diagnosis

The radionics practitioner 'tunes' in to his patient by studying charts and dials and turning knobs on his black box.

Some radionics practitioners claim to be able to provide a postal diagnostic service. They invite patients to send in samples of hair – and they then write back with advice.

The provision of treatment

Some radionics practitioners claim that they can 'treat' their patients simply by using their black boxes to beam out corrective radiations. Others prefer to use other treatment techniques. Some of the remedies used by radionics practitioners include: biochemic tissue salts, Bach flower remedies, vitamin supplements and homoeopathy.

Research

I have been unable to find any research evidence to show that radionics is of value.

Qualifications and training for radionics

It is possible to follow a course of radionics training.

Dangers

I know of no specific dangers associated with radionics.

The uses of radionics

I know of none.

REBIRTHING

The background

Those who practise 'rebirthing' or 'birth enactment' believe that many patterns of human behaviour and some illnesses are produced by the traumas associated with birth. They claim that it is possible to eradicate these mental traumas by guiding the patient back into the womb and reliving the whole experience.

To make a diagnosis

No diagnosis is involved in rebirthing.

The provision of treatment

Rebirthing is stage managed in a number of different ways. Some practitioners simply guide their patients back into the womb by visualization techniques (see page 177). Some use deep breathing exercises. Occasionally practitioners used the drug LSD. Sometimes patients are encouraged to adopt the foetal position while they are being 'rebirthed'. Perhaps the most dramatic rebirthing technique is to provide a tunnel of blankets for the patient to deliver himself or herself through.

Research

I have been unable to find any research evidence to prove that this technique is of real value.

Qualifications and training for rebirthing

Rebirthing is practised and taught by a wide variety of 'therapists'.

Dangers

It is possible that a patient could acquire severe mental problems by following this technique. (See also the technique 'regression' described under *Hypnotherapy*, page 119.)

The uses of rebirthing

I do not believe that 'rebirthing' has any uses.

REFLEXOLOGY

The background

Although most practitioners claim that reflexology or reflex zone therapy was practised several thousand years ago by both the Chinese and the Egyptians modern reflexology was first introduced in the 1920s by an American physician called William Fitzgerald.

Fitzgerald claimed to have discovered a relationship between ten different parts or zones of the body and ten matching zones on the feet. There are various different schools of reflexology in existence today but most base their findings on Dr Fitzgerald's work.

According to Fitzgerald all the glands, organs and major nerves of the body have corresponding nerve endings in the toes and feet. The right foot represents the right-hand side of the body and the left foot represents the left-hand side of the body. An imaginary line drawn half-way down the foot approximates to the waist. The big toe represents the head and brain and the little toe represents the sinuses.

Illness, claimed Fitzgerald, is caused by the accumulation of crystalline deposits around those nerve endings in the feet.

To make a diagnosis

In order to make a diagnosis reflexologists examine their patients' feet carefully and thoroughly, massaging and probing every inch of the sole of each foot. They claim that every corn and callous and sore place denotes some significant problem elsewhere (they fail to take into account the influence of ill-fitting shoes and socks).

The provision of treatment

Once having diagnosed a problem, reflexologists claim that they can treat it by massaging the appropriate part of the appropriate foot.

They warn that their technique is so powerful that it can unsettle the hormonal balance of the body if over-used and that patients with diabetes or thyroid disorders can find that their disease is sent temporarily out of control. They claim to be able to help patients with all sorts of problems but generally seem to believe that their skills are best suited to the treatment of the following: asthma, backache, poor circulation, tension, stiffness, sinus troubles, dandruff, infertility, stammering, multiple sclerosis, irregular periods and piles.

Cynics will note that the only thing all these disorders have in common is that they do tend to come and go by themselves.

Research

There is, inevitably, some anecdotal evidence to support the reflexologists. I know of no independent scientific evidence to support these claims.

Qualifications and training for reflexology

There are special schools and colleges where reflexology is taught.

Dangers

Reflexology is unlikely to lead to any specific problems.

The uses of reflexology

A good foot massage is extremely soothing (and, surprisingly perhaps, does not tickle). The feet are well-endowed with nerve endings and they are frequently abused by too much walking and standing. By skilfully massaging a patient's feet a reflexologist will be able to soothe and relax troubled muscles and tissues – as well as calming and relaxing the patient with careful concern and thoughtful conversation.

A reflexology session is likely to last between thirty minutes and one hour and it would be surprising if most patients did not feel better after lying down for that length of time.

The real weakness of reflexology must, however, be its failure to take into account other pressures and forces which affect the condition of the foot.

ROLFING

The background

Rolfing is a complex manipulative technique developed in the 1940s and 1950s by the late Ida Rolf, a Swiss biochemist. The Rolfer tries to change the physical alignment of the body in order to improve the physiological and psychological functioning of the body.

Rolf, like Wilhelm Reich and F. M. Alexander, believed that physical misalignment can lead to all sorts of problems. She believed that a body's relationship to gravity influences its wellbeing and vitality and argued that in order to benefit fully from the remarkable force of gravity a man or woman should operate through a straight vertical plane.

To make a diagnosis

Rolfing is essentially a therapeutic procedure.

The provision of treatment

The aim of 'rolfing' is to realign the plastic, malleable structure of the body. The aim is to support the energy field of man with the energy field of gravity.

In practice rolfing involves the massage of the tissues to correct all deviations from the vertical alignment of the skeleton. Ten one-hour sessions are needed and the pressure and kneading of the muscles and tissues can be painful. Those who practise rolfing claim that patients may be taller afterwards and will move with more grace and symmetry.

Research

I know of no independent research to substantiate the

claims made by those who practise rolfing.

Qualifications and training for rolfing

It is possible to follow a course in rolfing.

Dangers

If rolfing is done on a patient in a weakened state – suffering from cancer or an infection, for example – it is possible that muscles, bones and/or joints could be damaged.

The uses of rolfing

I know of no specific conditions for which I would recommend rolfing. The Alexander Technique seems a more sensible approach to posture problems and ordinary massage is probably just as good as rolfing for muscle disorders.

SHIATSU

The background

Shiatsu – which literally means finger pressure – is the modern merging of acupuncture and traditional Chinese massage techniques. Instead of using needles (as in acupuncture) the shiatsu practitioner uses his fingers to exert pressure and bring the body back into balance.

Acupressure techniques are a 'mass market' version of shiatsu.

To make a diagnosis

The shiatsu practitioner makes his diagnosis after taking a good history from the patient.

The provision of treatment

Shiatsu massage is given either for specific problems or in order to improve the general health of a patient.

The shiatsu practitioner puts a considerable amount of pressure on the specific points of the patient's body that he 'attacks'. He uses his thumbs a good deal and may even use his elbows to direct pressure to certain areas of the body.

Research

I know of no scientific research to show that shiatsu is of specific value. There is, however, a considerable amount of research evidence to show the value of acupuncture (see page 31).

Qualifications and training for shiatsu

It is possible to take a training course in shiatsu – although, as always, the quality of teaching varies as much as the quality of the students.

Dangers

As long as shiatsu is not performed on inflamed, infected, damaged or cancerous areas then there should be no real dangers. However, it is important that shiatsu is not practised where further damage to muscles, bones and joints may occur.

The uses of shiatsu

Shiatsu is probably of some value in the treatment of the sort of conditions for which acupuncture (and acupressure) are of value.

SILVA METHOD

The background

The Silva Method (also known as Silva Mind Control) was developed in the 1950s by Jose Silva, a Mexican American who developed his techniques after exploring a number of methods of maximizing human potential (including hypnotism, positive thinking, meditation and biofeedback).

To make a diagnosis

The Silva Method is not a diagnostic technique.

The provision of treatment

The aim of treatment with the Silva Method is to relax the patient thoroughly by use of meditation and then to use the abilities which become available at this deeper level to strengthen and reinforce the patient's urge for change and self-improvement.

Research

There is a considerable amount of evidence available to show that meditation has a positive effect (see page 139). I know of no specific research evidence to show that the Silva Method is superior to other forms of meditation and self-improvement.

Qualifications and training for the Silva Method

Those who teach the Silva Method are trained by the organization which promotes the technique.

Dangers

I know of no specific dangers associated with the Silva Method.

The uses of the Silva Method

See Meditation (page 140).

TENS MACHINE

The background

Using electricity to relieve pain is nothing new. Ancient Egyptians and Hippocrates are said to have used electricity and in AD46 a Roman physician called Scribonius Largus is credited with having claimed to be able to cure headaches with the energy produced by an electric torpedo fish.

After that promising start the role of electricity in medicine was forgotten for the best part of two thousand years. Then in the middle part of the nineteenth century it once again became fashionable to talk about electricity as a pain-relieving aid. All sorts of wonderful gadgets were put on the market, and excessive claims were made by the manufacturers.

The real value of electricity as a pain reliever was really only discovered fairly recently, however, and came about after the gate control theory was widely accepted.

The gate control theory suggests that when the skin or tissues are damaged, messages carrying information about the injury travel towards the brain along two quite separate sets of nerve fibres. The larger fibres carry messages about sensations other than pain and the smaller nerve fibres carry pain messages. The messages travelling along the large fibres tend to arrive at the spinal cord before the messages travelling along the smaller fibres and, if there are enough non-painful sensations travelling, the pain messages won't be able to get through.

The gate control theory enabled scientists to explain all sorts of natural phenomena that had up until then been a mystery to physiologists. It became clear, for example, that when we rub a sore spot we are increasing the number of non-painful messages travelling towards the spinal cord's nerve gateway. If you knock your elbow you'll automatically reach to rub the spot because subconsciously you know that by rubbing the area you'll be able to cut down the amount of pain that you feel.

Having realized just how rubbing a sore spot can relieve pain, the next step was for scientists to come up with a way of stimulating the passage of non-painful sensations quite automatically. They had the idea of using electricity to produce the necessary stimulus.

When the theory was first put into practice in the late 1960s doctors suggested that the electricity should be introduced into the body through electrodes surgically implanted into the spine. Although that did seem to work, the fact that it involved a surgical operation (though only a minor one) limited the usefulness and availability of the procedure.

The next development made the whole concept much more readily available. It was discovered that all nerves within an inch or two of the surface of the skin can be stimulated by electrodes which are simply stuck on to the skin.

And that was exactly what the next teams of researchers started doing. They started giving patients pocket-sized battery-operated stimulators which sent out a continuous series of electrical pulses and which could transmit those pulses into the large nerves of the body via silicone electrodes stuck on to the skin with a special conducting paste. And it worked.

Moreover, it was found that Transcutaneous Electrical Nerve Stimulation (it quickly became known as TENS) didn't just stimulate the passage of sensory impulses designed to inhibit the passage of pain impulses; it also stimulated the body to start producing its own pain-relieving hormones, the endorphins.

Obviously, the next step was to start conducting experiments to see how effective TENS was. And during the last decade a number of impressive projects have shown without doubt that TENS is extremely effective in relieving pain.

To make a diagnosis

TENS is a treatment device and does not involve making a diagnosis.

The provision of treatment

TENS machines can be bought commercially although they are sometimes 'prescribed' by medical advisers.

There are two variables with every TENS device: the strength of the electrical pulse being produced by the machine and the position where the electrodes are applied.

Getting the level of stimulation right is fairly straightforward. All you have to do is increase the stimulation until it produces pain and then turn it down until it is comfortable. When you feel a pleasant and acceptable tingling, the machine is 'set'.

Finding the right place for the electrodes is more difficult. Some machines have two electrodes, others have four simply to give you double the chance to stimulate the appropriate nerves. Most experts recommend that you begin by placing the electrodes on the points of greatest tenderness. If stimulating them for thirty minutes or so doesn't help relieve your pain then you should simply move the electrodes over the painful area until you find a spot where they do work. Or you can try pressing your skin with your fingers until you find tender spots and then stick your electrodes over those points.

The TENS device suppresses pain not only at the time but also, it seems, long after the machine has been switched off. Many patients find that they can free themselves of pain more or less completely by using their device as little as two or three times a week. Others find that they need to keep their device in place permanently and use it virtually all the time.

Research

In a study conducted with patients suffering from rheumatoid arthritis it was found that the TENS equipment produced pain relief in up to 95 per cent of patients. In other experiments it was found that TENS even managed to produce relief in patients who had received no relief from any other pain-relieving techniques. Dr John Bonica, one of the world's leading experts on pain relief, has said that TENS machines provide short-term relief for 65–80 per cent of all pain patients and long-term relief for between 30 and 50 per cent of patients. According to Professor John Thompson, Professor of Pharmacology at the University of Newcastle upon Tyne, who is consultant clinical pharmacologist for the Newcastle Health Authority and consultant in charge at the pain relief clinic at the Royal Victoria Infirmary in Newcastle, short-term improvement after using TENS may be between 80 and 90 per cent with a very respectable 35 per cent of patients still benefiting from pain relief after two years' use. It has been shown that the TENS machine is good for relieving low back pain, phantom limb pain, arthritis of all kinds, cancer pain and the pain that sometimes develops after herpes. A large study done in Sweden has shown that TENS is the only painkiller required by 70 per cent of women in labour. It works well for patients recovering from surgery too.

Qualifications and training for TENS machines

Anyone can use a TENS machine. There is no need for training or qualifications.

Dangers

Apart from the fact that TENS shouldn't be used by pregnant women (because it is always wise to be cautious if you are pregnant) or by people who have a heart pacemaker and that you shouldn't try to use one if you're driving, and that you shouldn't use it around the eyes, there aren't really any dangers or problems with it. The commonest side effect seems to be a slight skin rash caused by the jelly used to stick the electrodes to the skin.

The uses of TENS machines

TENS seems to work best with persistent and fairly stable pains; headaches, stiff necks, backaches, joint pains and period pains, for example, rather than pains that are sudden, acute or shooting. And second, even though TENS doesn't always cut out pain completely, it very often relieves it enough to enable a disabled or bedbound patient to become an active member of the community again. If a TENS device can make the difference between lying in bed and living a fairly normal life then the investment has to be worth while.

TENS devices are safe, effective and economical. Their ultimate advantage is that they work not by attacking the body but by stimulating the body's own pain-relieving mechanisms.

URINE THERAPY

The background

Urine therapy is one of those strange medical disciplines that tends to become popular for a while, disappear for a few hundred years and then suddenly reappear again for no very good reason.

The theory behind urine therapy is that although urine is usually 96 per cent water it does contain all the salts and hormones that the body needs. The people who practise this strange form of treatment argue that urine can be used to treat genital herpes, cancer, heart disease, kidney problems, gall stones, multiple sclerosis, diabetes, testicular problems, tooth decay, eye disorders, stomach ulcers, burns, bites and open wounds.

To make a diagnosis

Urine therapy is a therapy and there is no allied diagnostic skill (although in the past some 'experts' have claimed that they can make a wide range of diagnoses simply by smelling or tasting urine samples).

The provision of treatment

If your problem is a superficial one (a cut or a burn, for example) then it is suggested that you treat yourself by pouring urine over the affected area.

But if the problem is an internal one then you are advised to drink the urine. Your own is probably best but aficionados of this particular type of therapy are usually quite happy to drink anyone else's that happens to be available. Nor do they mind if urine is infected, discoloured or full of blood.

Research

I know of no research to substantiate the claims made by those who practise urine therapy.

Qualifications and training for urine therapy

I know of no training courses for urine therapists.

Dangers

Drinking urine is a potentially dangerous practice. In small quantities urine is unlikely to do any harm at all. Drunk regularly it could prove extremely damaging.

The uses of urine therapy

Urine therapy is a bizarre and unnatural form of treatment. Urine is full of waste materials discharged from the body because the body doesn't need them. The kidneys filter the blood regularly in order to remove electrolytes that are accumulating in excessive quantities and urine production is organized to ensure that any substances that look as if they are likely to build up in dangerous quantities are discharged from the body as quickly as possible.

Drinking urine is as sensible as breathing stale air.

VEGETARIANISM

The background

Those who recommend a vegetarian diet usually claim that it is more 'natural' than a mixed diet.

This is nonsense.

The vegetarian foods eaten by our ancestors a few million years ago contained neither cereals nor pulses. Our real ancestors lived on leaves, fruits and nuts – and some meat. The cereals that vegetarians eat are just as unnatural as the types of meat that the domestication of animals has made available. And while it is perfectly true that much of the meat that we eat these days is far too fatty that is hardly an argument for cutting out meat completely.

To make a diagnosis

Vegetarianism is a way of life, rather than an aid to diagnosis.

The provision of treatment

Vegetarianism is a way of life, rather than a form of treatment.

Research

The evidence shows that, far from making themselves healthier, vegetarians are just as likely to develop (and die of) heart disease as those who eat whatever they fancy. There is also evidence to suggest that some types of cancer are commoner among those who stick to a vegetarian diet, that vegetarians can develop vitamin and mineral shortages and that it is all too easy to get your food intake out of balance if you stick to one particular type of diet.

Vegans (who take no food of animal origin – including milk, eggs and cheese) are particularly vulnerable to deficiency disorders.

It has been said that putting a small child on an exclusion diet is a form of child abuse. The human body is designed for a mixed diet and any diet that concentrates on one particular type of food to the exclusion of all others is unnatural and unhealthy.

Qualifications and training for vegetarianism

There is no need for special training to become a vegetarian.

Dangers

Vitamin and mineral deficiencies can occur (see above).

The uses of vegetarianism

A vegetarian diet is defensible on moral grounds but not on health grounds.

VISUALIZATION

The background

The relationship between imagination and reality is closer than you think. And it is a relationship that has been acknowledged and accepted for a long time. William Shakespeare wrote that, 'There is nothing good or bad, but thinking makes it so.' And more recently the philosopher William James announced that in his opinion, too, human beings could, by changing the inner attitudes of their minds change the outer aspects of their lives, and thereby control their own destinies.

Only in the last few years, however, have these philosophical conclusions been translated into practical reality. While the majority of physicians and surgeons around the world have continued to concentrate on using knives, poisons, electricity, chemicals and radiation to attack disease and disorder (forgetting that the battleground, the human body, is often as vulnerable to the weapons being employed as the disease itself), a small but persistent number of researchers has continued to experiment with techniques involving the imagination. It is a weapon that is both simple and sophisticated, commonplace and unique, remarkably easy to use and yet far more powerful than any other available tool.

As is well known, the human imagination can prove destructive and damaging. If a man thinks he has a cancer developing there is a very good chance indeed that he will develop a cancer. If a woman thinks she is going to lose her baby the chances of her losing her baby are greatly enhanced. If a man thinks he is going to have a heart attack, he will probably have a heart attack. If a woman thinks she is likely to die, she will probably die.

It is this power of the imagination over the body that accounts for the strengths of the voodoo priest and the African witchdoctor. It is the same power that underpins the doctor's ability to convince his patients of his own infallibility. It is the same power that explains the placebo effect and the ability of an untrained healer to conquer pain and disease with nothing more mysterious than his own hands.

In the past the power of the imagination has been used almost exclusively as a method of augmenting the unnatural skills of the interventionist. The general practitioner and the hospital specialist use their patients' imaginations when telling them that the prescription they are providing will banish their symptoms. The homoeopath, the hypnotherapist, the acupuncturist and the herbalist all use the imagination to augment and enhance their own limited technical skills.

When the professional suggests to the patient that he will get better the patient's imagination responds by triggering the release of natural pain-relieving hormones – the endorphins. And when the patient duly gets better the professional usually takes the credit.

Recently, however, it has become clear that in order to harness the power of his imagination the patient does not necessarily need the help of a medical professional. He needs only to believe in the power of his imagination in order to benefit from its potential strength. He has to learn a few simple, creative 'tricks' in order to harness these powers but the basic requirement, the fundamental essential prerequisite, is that he believes.

To make a diagnosis

Visualization does not involve making a diagnosis.

The provision of treatment

When you fall ill and need to use the powers of your imagination to help you combat very real symptoms, there are a number of simple ways in which you can stimulate your imagination to help you – ways in which you can use 'visualization' to speed your recovery.

1 Always think of yourself getting better and try to see yourself fully recovered, doing all the things you would normally do. If you develop the early symptoms of a cold and you visualize yourself snuffling away in bed and missing all sorts of important appointments, you'll probably end up in bed with a terrible cold – missing all sorts of important appointments.

If, however, you see yourself recovering from your cold after a few hours' mild snuffling, the cold symptoms will disappear and you won't need to miss any appointments at all. Naturally, I'm not promising that you can stay healthy all the time simply by seeing yourself as healthy – some genuine problems will require outside help – but minor troubles such as coughs, colds and aches and pains can often be defeated in this simple way. And even when your imagination on its own cannot defeat illness, it is much better to have it working on your side than to have it contributing strength to your illness. At the very worst, your imagination will help minimize the length of time that you are ill.

2   Never think of any disease as being strong or powerful. Always think of your body as being stronger than any attacking force. If you have an infection of any kind think of the infective organisms as being evil, but weak, homeless, lonely and frightened. And think of your body as a tower of strength. If you have a cancer think of it as an uncertain intruder, struggling to survive. If you think of a cancer or infection as a 'being', think of it as weak and weedy, having a hacking cough and terrible skin.

3   Try leaving your body if you are suffering from pain or some specific illness. Decide that you'll move to a far corner of the room and settle yourself down to help heal your body. Imagine that you can see yourself from the front, the side, the back and from above. Leave the pain or the illness behind. Now see your body being helped by teams of skilled and dedicated doctors. See the experts removing the disease and eradicating the pain. Visualize the disease as a pile of rubbish that simply needs to be cleaned out and carried away. Imagine that the pain in your body is being transmitted along special wires and try to see the doctors cutting those wires. Don't re-enter your body until you are satisfied that the doctors have done as much as they can for the time being.

4   If you are being treated with drugs of any kind imagine each tablet or capsule as being full of special miniature fighting forces. Imagine those forces being released in your stomach, finding their way into your blood stream and travelling around your body fighting the disease that is affecting you. Imagine the white blood cells in your body fighting also on your behalf. Think of your fighting forces as cowboys, as cavalry, as spacemen or as medieval knights of the Round Table. It really doesn't

matter how you use your imagination as long as you use it in a positive and dramatic way and as long as you pick images in which you can believe and have faith.

Research

In an experiment conducted in Australia in 1983 researchers took a large group of people who had absolutely nothing in common apart from the fact that none of them had ever played basketball before. After being allowed to spend one day throwing basketballs through a hoop the volunteers were divided into three separate groups.

The first group were to play absolutely no basketball for a month. They were told not even to think about basketball. The second group were told to practise every day. And the third group were told to spend ten minutes a day imagining that they were throwing balls into a basket.

At the end of the one month experiment the people in the first group were no better at basketball than they had been at the start of the whole exercise. However, the other two groups had improved by closely similar amounts. The players who had been spending their time out on the court throwing basketballs through hoops had improved by 24 per cent. And the players who had been spending ten minutes a day imagining that they had been throwing basketballs through hoops had improved by 23 per cent.

Even more impressive has been the work done in America by Dr Carl Simonton and his wife. For a number of years now they have been teaching patients how to cope with cancer by using their imaginations. The theory is that if the imagination can have a destructive effect, it can also have a positive effect. If people can give themselves cancer by negative thinking they should be able to protect themselves against cancer and maybe even cure themselves of cancer by positive thinking. If people can give themselves cancer by being miserable and sad, perhaps they can help get themselves better by being happy and cheerful. In the first years of their experiment the Simontons have found that their patients have lived, on average, more than a year longer than patients who were not encouraged to use their minds to help fight their disease.

Qualifications and training for visualization

There is no need for any training or qualifications, either to practise or to teach visualisation techniques.

Dangers

None.

The uses of visualization

Some of this may sound alarmingly simple. But that is only because we have been trained to think of medical technology as having all the answers and of our bodies as being fundamentally weak and fragile. And yet the evidence shows that our bodies have powers that we have consistently underestimated. Our minds can make our bodies ill. But they can also keep them healthy – and make us well again.

VITAMIN THERAPY

The background

The sale of vitamin and mineral supplements is now big business. Encouraged to believe that they need specific supplements, both in order to fight off specific diseases and in order to retain good health, many thousands of people take huge amounts of pills every day. The size of the market tends to grow each year since once a new customer has been recruited the vitamin salesman can usually depend upon a more or less permanent sale. Consumers acquire a psychological addiction to their tablets and often take them for many years.

The manufacture and sale of vitamin supplements is nothing new, of course. Back in 1923 the editors of the *British Medical Journal* were so worried about what they saw as a relatively new phenomenon that they ran an article entitled, 'The Vitamin Content of Certain Proprietary Preparations' written by, among others, the then professor of pharmacology at the University of London.

The authors concluded:

> Our experiments confirm what other workers on vitamins have emphasised – namely, that under normal conditions of life an adequate supply of vitamins can be easily ensured by including in the diet a suitable amount of protective foods such as milk, butter, green vegetables and fruit and that no advantage is to be gained by trying to obtain these substances in the form of drugs.

That was fifty years ago but the people selling vitamins have continued to promote their products with all sorts of pseudo-scientific arguments. With the aid of a handful of scientists and one or two publicity-seeking eccentrics the vitamin industry has continued to create and then satisfy a series of artificial needs.

One of the most successful marketing strategies was to announce that vitamin C could be used to help fight off colds. Although this suggestion was entirely discredited back in the mid 1970s by a series of clinical trials which showed conclusively that there was no scientific basis in the belief that vitamin C supplements would provide protection against such infections, there are still many people who believe the advertising they read. In one of the most damning pieces of evidence – published in the *Journal of the American Medical Association* – details were given of a trial in which marine recruits were each given 2 gm doses of vitamin C in an attempt to stop them getting colds. The researchers found that the pills had absolutely no protective effect whatsoever.

To make a diagnosis

One or two authors have suggested that it is possible to diagnose vitamin deficiency by examining and recording signs and symptoms of ill health.

The provision of treatment

There are scores of companies and shops now promoting vitamin supplements for a wide range of different conditions. Sometimes vitamin supplements are 'prescribed' but more commonly they are distributed on a retail basis.

Research

The available research shows that vitamin supplements are of no value – unless the individual concerned is already vitamin deficient. According to a report published in the *Drug and Therapeutics Bulletin*, May 1984, only one or two people in every 1,000 suffer from vitamin deficiency. And they, of course, need properly prescribed vitamin supplements as well as decent dietary advice in order to ensure that their problem does not persist.

Qualifications and training for vitamin therapy

Vitamins are promoted and recommended by many individuals – most of whom have no specific training or qualifications.

Dangers

What most vitamin suppliers fail to tell their customers is that taking extra vitamin tablets can be quite dangerous. There is an over-whelming amount of evidence available to show that the people promoting vitamin supplements have probably done more harm than good. Too many vitamin supplements can cause depression, anxiety and a whole range of diseases. When taken in excessive amounts vitamins can kill. Some observers have noted that diseases caused by taking too many vitamins are now more common than disorders caused by vitamin deficiency.

Vitamin A taken in excess can produce anorexia, drowsiness, irritability, hair loss, headache and skin problems. Too much vitamin C can cause kidney problems and can affect growing bones. In addition people who have been taking high doses of vitamin C and suddenly cut down their intake can develop rebound scurvy. Vitamin D in high doses can cause irreversible damage to the eyes and the kidneys. It can also cause fits, comas and muscular weakness. Vitamin E in high doses can produce spontaneous bleeding, can reduce sexual function and can also produce headaches, eye problems and stomach disorders.

The real tragedy is that many of the problems caused by taking too many vitamins are treated as vitamin deficiencies by the people concerned (usually following the inevitably biased advice of the people trying to sell more vitamins) with dreadful consequences.

Undoubtedly worried lest the vitamin market eventually collapse under the weight of evidence showing the uselessness and danger of supplements, the vitamin industry has in the last few years begun to spend huge amounts of money promoting mineral supplements. At least nine trace elements – iron, zinc, copper, manganese, cobalt, chromium, selenium, molybdenum and iodine – are required in tiny amounts for good health. The problem is that no one really knows what these elements are needed for, nor what quantities are required. What we do know is that when taken in excess the minerals can cause just as many problems as their absence can create. Some manufacturers promoting mineral supplements are behaving remarkably irresponsibly and risking their customers' health by publishing astonishing recommendations in promotional literature.

The uses of vitamin therapy

Most of the claims made for vitamins are entirely untrue. And many of the rest are based on flimsy, disputable or extremely rocky evidence. The plain truth is that taking vitamin supplements blindly is interventionist medicine at its very worst. It is about as far from holistic medicine as electro-convulsive therapy or destructive brain surgery.

YOGA

The background

Yoga is a discipline which originated in the East and which combines meditation, gentle physical exercise and a healthy lifestyle. It is a form of preventive medicine designed to keep both the body and the mind as fit as possible.

To make a diagnosis

There are no diagnostic skills associated with yoga.

The provision of treatment

Yoga is a form of preventive medicine – rather than a specific therapy.

Research

I know of no specific research to show the superiority of yoga to other forms of meditation and relaxation.

Qualifications and training for yoga

There are many training courses for yoga. Some are undoubtedly excellent. I have, however discovered one yoga teacher training course available by post which surprises me.

At the end of this correspondence course 'a certificate of completion' is issued once students advise the course tutor that they have completed their studies satisfactorily.

It is difficult to imagine a less arduous educational requirement.

Dangers

I know of no specific hazards that are associated with yoga.

The uses of yoga

Yoga is usually (and to a certain extent unfairly) associated with uncomfortable, unlikely and sometimes downright impossible positions. Some would-be students are put off because they feel that they are not lithe enough, supple enough or slender enough to don a leotard and show their thighs in public. The undoubtedly quasi-religious aspects of the discipline do frighten some people off.

However, despite these disadvantages yoga undoubtedly satisfies many people's needs for a routine that will lead to a healthier life and lifestyle.

THE END

THE PATIENT'S COMPANION
by Dr. Vernon Coleman

'Definitely a worthwhile buy'
Woman's Own

'. . . a useful reference tool for the medicine cupboard'
The Times

'A mine of highly readable, well-organised information'
Company

The Patient's Companion was first published as *The Good Medicine Guide*, and has now been completely revised and updated for this new paperback edition.

Dr. Vernon Coleman is one of Britain's bestselling writers on medicine and this excellent reference book has been written to help everyone to get the very best health care for themselves and their families.

* how to read a prescription
* what to stock in your medicine cupboard
* what to do when someone dies
* what to take to hospital
* what a form FP 95 is (and 35 other forms that doctors hand out to patients)
* how to leave your body to a medical school
* how to change your doctor
* how to seek advice when going abroad
* what vaccinations you and your child need

0 552 12734 5

BODYPOWER
by Dr. Vernon Coleman

This book, contains a single, simple, sensational secret.

A secret whose importance has been disguised, suppressed or merely ignored not only by the doctors, drug companies, administrators and politicians who control Western medicine, but also by the practitioners of alternative remedies – herbalists and hypnotists, ocupuncturists and gurus, with their complicated, and often expensive, methods.

Your body is equipped with an enormous range of subtle and sophisticated feedback mechanisms. Some – like those designed to ensure that your body temperature is kept at the right level – help to protect you against changes in your environment. Some – like the device which raises your body temperature to intolerable levels for infecting or organisms – are there to fight off disease. Many are given the job of regulating what you eat and drink according to what you need.

These internal mechanisms are so effective that in at least ninety per cent of illnesses you will be able to recover without any form of medical treatment. BODYPOWER tells you about them, reveals why they have often become ineffective in modern life, shows how to use them in combating a wide variety of illnesses – and teaches you to recognize when you *must* have professional help.

BODYPOWER is a remarkable system, developed by a widely experienced doctor, to help you benefit from your body's extraordinary ability to heal itself.

0 552 99262 3

ADDICTS & ADDICTIONS
by Dr. Vernon Coleman

'Dr Coleman has produced an excellent plain-man's guide to a phenomenon both puzzling and horrifying . . . his book will be most welcomed by friends and relatives of addicts'
Yorkshire Evening Post

Addiction can wreck homes, destroy careers and ruin lives, yet for years families of addicts have had to shoulder alone a burden that the rest of society has chosen to ignore. **Addicts and Addictions** offers help, guidance and information to those concerned, caring people. It seeks also to help the people who are addicted in some way. And it will be of vital use to those whose job it is to look after them.

Addiction in all its many forms is no longer just a problem that affects an unfortunate and eccentric few. It is the epidemic of the twentieth century, exploding so fast that there is barely a family in the country that is not affected.

Dr Vernon Coleman takes a simple, straightforward look at the different types of addiction, including people who rely excessively on gambling, exercise and work. He describes how you can recognise an addict; what the dangers are of long-term use, and of withdrawal; and how addicts and their addictions should be treated.

·Alcohol·Amphetamines·Barbiturates·Benzodia-zepines·Cannabis·Cocaine·Glue and Solvents·Heroin·LSD·Tobacco·Exercise·Food·Gambling·Work·

0 552 99238 0

STRESS WITHOUT DISTRESS
by Hans Selye

'Hans Selye knows more about stress than any other scientist. Here, taking off his lab coat and speaking simply to all of us, he offers a lifetime of learning about how to survive in a pressure-ridden society.

STRESS WITHOUT DISTRESS is not only a helpful book. It is thoughtful, wise, and moral in the best sense of that word Alvin Toffler, author of FUTURE SHOCK.

'Stress is the spice of life', says Dr Selye. Without it you would be a vegetable – or dead. Then why can stress be destructive, causing ulcers, heart disease, and so many other ailments of modern society?

To those and other vital questions about health and self-fulfilment, Dr Selye in STRESS WITHOUT DISTRESS offers reassuring answers, based on a lifetime of pioneering biological research.

He explains the physiological mechanisms of stress and offers specific advice on avoiding stress that is harmful. He tells you what to do if you're baffled by a problem, why procrastination is dangerous, how to enjoy leisure, why aimlessness causes distress. He discusses the concept of work as rewarding and satisfying play, and the relationship between work, stress and aging.

STRESS WITHOUT DISTRESS shows how you can increase your potential in a practical and natural way without endangering your health with harmful stress factors.

0 552 13002 8

HOMEOPHATHIC MEDICINE AT HOME
by Maesimund B. Panos M.D. and Jane Heimlich

Alternative Medicine the natural way in your own home

HOW TO CHOOSE AND USE HOMEOPATHIC
TREATMENT

Homeopathy has long been recognised as an effective alternative to modern medical techniques, with the bonus that homeopathic remedies are non-toxic, safe for children and pregnant women and do not cause side-effects.

HOMEOPATHIC MEDICINE AT HOME is a comprehensive and practical guide to self-help homeopathy and tells you how to treat minor ailments, deal with emergencies and how to prescribe for yourself and your family.

- Your Home Remedy Kit
- What to do for Accidents
- A Happier Baby with Homeopathic Care
- How to Prevent and Treat Colds, Coughs, Ear-ache, Indigestion
- Your Growing Child
- What Homeopathy can do for Women
- Keeping your Pets Healthy

0 552 99244 5

NON FICTION AVAILABLE FROM PATHWAY

The prices shown below were correct at the time of going to press. However Transworld Publishers reserve the right to show new retail prices on covers which may differ from those previously advertised in the text or elsewhere.

ORDER FORM

All Corgi/Bantam Books are available at your bookshop or newsagent, or can be ordered direct from the following address:

Corgi/Bantam Books,
Cash Sales Department,
P.O. Box 11, Falmouth, Cornwall TR10 9EN.

Please send a cheque or postal order (no currency) and allow 60p for postage and packing for the first book plus 25p for the second book and 15p for each additional book ordered up to a maximum charge of £1.90 in UK.

B.F.P.O. customers please allow 60p for the first book, 25p for the second book plus 15p per copy for the next 7 books, thereafter 9p per book.

Overseas customers, including Eire, please allow £1.25 for postage and packing for the first book, 75p for the second book, and 28p for each subsequent title ordered.

NAME (Block Letters) ....

ADDRESS...

....